Legal aspects of health and safety

2nd Edition

Other titles in the series include

Legal Aspects of Consent 2nd edition
Legal Aspects of Death
Legal Aspects of Medicines 2nd edition
Legal Aspects of Patient Confidentiality 2nd edition
Legal Aspects of Pain Management 2nd edition

Note

Healthcare practice and knowledge are constantly changing and developing as new research and treatments, changes in procedures, drugs and equipment become available.

The author and publishers have, as far as is possible, taken care to confirm that the information complies with the latest standards of practice and legislation.

Legal Aspects of Health and Safety

2nd Edition

by

Bridgit Dimond

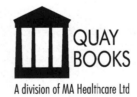

QUAY BOOKS

A division of MA Healthcare Ltd

Quay Books Division, MA Healthcare Ltd, St Jude's Church, Dulwich Road, London
SE24 0PB

British Library Cataloguing-in-Publication Data
A catalogue record is available for this book

ISBN-10: 1-85642-417-0
ISBN-13: 978-1-85642-417-2

Edited by Jessica Anderson

Cover design by Louise Cowburn, Fonthill Creative

Associate Publisher: Thu Nguyen

Printed by CLE, Huntingdon, Cambridgeshire

Contents

s of
care.
cation
fety in

nanagers,
entatives.
law can be
l system are
ncyclopaedic
asic principles
g up the further
about health and
is never finished
e amendments, bu
s can develop thei

Bridgit Dimon
November, 200

v

Preface to the 1st Edition

Like the other books in this series, this text follows the publication of a seri~
articles in the *British Journal of Nursing* on health and safety law in health~
Those articles, revisited and updated, form the basis of a concise publi~
covering the main concerns which arise in the law relating to health and s~
the National Health Service.

This book is intended for all health professionals, health service ~
professional associations and trade unions, patient groups and their repr~
Each chapter uses a situation to illustrate the relevant laws so that the~
explained in a practical jargon-free way. The basic facts of the leg~
briefly set out in the first chapter. The book does not pretend to be ~
in its coverage, rather it is intended to introduce readers to the ~
which apply and the sources of law, so that they can, by followi~
reading and websites provided, add to their knowledge. Writing~
safety law is like painting the bridge over the river Forth: it~
Changes in the statutory provisions and new cases require so~
hopefully this book will provide a baseline on which reade~
knowledge and understanding.

Preface to the 2nd Edition

Seven years is a long time in legal history and it is not surprising that this second edition contains many changes from the first. Not only is there the usual updating of statutes and statutory instruments including the first prosecution under the Corporate Manslaughter and Homicide Act and new cases amending rulings set in previous cases, but there are new NHS organisations such as the Care Quality Commission. In addition the Coalition Government is taking a fundamental review of health and safety legislation in the light of the Young Report *Common Sense Common Safety* 2010. The Health and Safety Commission merged with the Health and Safety Executive into a single body and further changes are taking place with the abolition of many quangos including the National Patient Safety Agency. New guidance has been given in many of the specific areas covered including health surveillance, COSHH regulations, manual handling, violence, bullying and stress.

It is hoped that this concise book will continue to provide a foundation for an understanding of the laws relating to health and safety within the context of health and social care.

Bridgit Dimond
June 2011

Acknowledgements

I should like to acknowledge my sincere thanks to Binkie Mais, my editor of the first edition, for her industrious and meticulous work, to Jessica Anderson editor of this second edition who has continued to maintain the high standard set by Binkie and to Bette Griffiths who prepared all the indexes with her usual care and skill.

CHAPTER 1

Introduction to the law

Scenario 1.1. Situation of ignorance

'The law says:...'

Amanda, a clinical nurse practitioner in the Accident and Emergency (A&E) Department is surprised one day when she is told by a staff nurse, that the law says that all patients in A&E Departments should be seen by a doctor before they leave the Department. Amanda questions this statement but does not know how to find the answer.

Introduction

This chapter provides an introduction to the main sources of law and the legal system. The following topics will be covered:

- Sources of law
- Human Rights Act
- Other international charters relating to health and safety
- Civil and criminal law
- Civil and criminal courts
- Public and private law
- Legal personnel
- Procedure in the civil courts
- Procedure in the criminal courts
- Accusatorial system
- Law and ethics
- Rules of Professional Conduct

Sources of law

Law derives from two main sources: statute law and the common law.

Statute law

Statute law is based on legislation passed through the agreed constitutional process. Legislation in the UK is formed by the introduction of a bill into either the House of Lords or House of Commons, sometimes by the Government, sometimes by a private member and follows through a recognised procedure by way of hearings, committee stages and report stage and, eventually, following agreement by both Houses and the signature of the Queen, becomes an Act of Parliament. The actual date it comes into force will either be set out in the Act itself or will be determined at a later date by statutory instrument (known as secondary legislation). The Act of Parliament may provide for powers to be delegated to Ministers and others to enacting detailed rules to supplement the Acts of Parliament. These are known as Statutory Instruments. They must be placed before Parliament before coming into effect. Since devolution, the Scottish Parliament has the right to enact legislation, within specified parameters; the Welsh Assembly has more powers since the Referendum held in 2011. The main legislation on health and safety is the Health and Safety at Work Act 1974 under which many regulations have been made in the form of statutory instruments. Some of the regulations result from European Community Directives.

As a consequence of its signing of the Treaty of Rome, and becoming a member of the European Community (EC), the United Kingdom is bound by the legislation of the EC. The EC Regulations have direct application to member states, unlike the EC Directives which must be incorporated into UK law to be effective. (This does not apply to their application to State authorities, where they are automatically binding.)

Common law

Decisions by judges in courts create what is known as the common law, case law or judge-made law. A recognised hierarchy of the courts determines which previous decisions are binding on courts hearing similar cases. The European Court of Justice, which is held in Luxembourg, can hear cases between member states on European laws, or applications by the domestic courts for a ruling on a point of law. A recognised system of reporting of judges' decisions ensures certainty over what was stated and the facts of the cases. The main principles that are set out in a case are known as the *ratio decidendi* (reasons for the decision). Other parts of a judge's speech, which are not considered to be part of the *ratio decidendi*, are known as *obiter dicta* (things said by the way). Only the *ratio decidendi* is directly binding on lower courts, but the *obiter dicta* may influence the decision of judges in later court cases. It may be possible for judges to 'distinguish' previous cases and not follow them on the grounds that the facts are significantly different. For example, before the Occupier's Liability Act 1984 was passed, which defined the liability of the occupier towards trespassers, the liability of the occupier to trespassers was based on decisions made by judges in disputes. Cases which involved harm to children where the occupier had been held liable, were held not to be binding on judges hearing cases involving adults, so that the occupier was held not to be liable to an adult trespasser. The earlier cases relating to children were 'distinguished'. Subsequently, legislation relating to the occupier's liability for trespassers was enacted in the Occupiers' Liability Act 1984 (*Chapter 9*).

Judges are, however, bound by statutes and if the result is an unsatisfactory situation, then this may be remedied by new amending legislation. If disputes in relation to the interpretation of the legislation arise, and the dispute is brought to court, then the specific section of the statute or paragraph of a statutory instrument has to be interpreted by the judge who will make a ruling. The decision may be appealed against by the party who has lost the case and eventually the Supreme Court may be called upon to make a decision. These decisions of the courts are known as precedents. Thus, law develops through a mix of statutory promulgation and common law decision making. The Human Rights Act 1998 (see below) takes precedence over other legislation, since a judge can make a declaration of incompatibility and can refer back to Parliament for reconsideration statutes which appear to infringe the articles set out in the European Convention of Human Rights.

Procedure for judicial review

The decisions of judicial and administrative bodies can be challenged by an application to the Queen's Bench Division for the decision or adjudication to be reviewed.

The Human Rights Act 1998

The European Convention for the Protection of Human Rights and Fundamental Freedoms (1950) provides protection for the fundamental rights and freedoms of all people. The UK was a signatory as were many European Countries which are not members of the European Community. Norway is a signatory to the European Commission on Human Rights but not a member of the European Community.

It is enforced through the European Commission and the European Court on Human Rights which meets in Strasbourg. However, following the passing of the Human Rights Act 1998 most of the articles are directly enforceable in the UK courts in relation to public authorities or organisations exercising functions of a public nature. Several articles of the European Convention relate to health and safety issues and they will be considered later in this book. For example, it has been alleged by some with disabilities that hoisting is contrary to their human rights under Article 3 and 14 (*Chapter 9*). In one case an employer argued that Section 40 of the Health and Safety at Work Act 1974, which placed a burden on an employer to show on a balance of probabilities that it had taken all reasonable precautions in fulfilling its statutory duties, was contrary to the presumption of innocence, and article 6(2) of the Convention (*Davies v. Health and Safety Executive* 2002). However, this argument was not accepted by the Court of Appeal which held that the 1974 Act was motivated by the need to protect public safety and the Act's regulatory nature meant that those operating within it had to conform to certain standards. In the field of health and safety it was acceptable to impose absolute duties on employers and it did not follow that a reverse burden on proof, within reasonable limits, would infringe article 6(2) (*Chapter 7*).

Other international charters relating to health

This country is also a signatory to, or has recognised, many other international charters which recognise rights in a variety of fields. These include: UN Convention on the Rights of the Child, the UN Convention on the Elimination of All Forms of Discrimination against Women, the Universal Declaration of Human Rights, the Declaration of Helsinki developed by the World Health Organization in 1964, recently amended in 2000 (relating to research practice). These Charters are not directly enforceable in this country, although some of their principles may be contained in statutes or common law, and reflected in guidance provided by the Department of Health and professional bodies and organisations.

Civil and criminal law

The civil law covers the law which governs disputes between citizens (including corporate bodies) or between citizens and the State. Contract law and the law of torts (civil wrongs excluding breach of contract), rights over property, marital disputes, wrongful exercise of power by a statutory authority, all come under the civil law. The sources of civil law are both statutory and the common law. Thus, the Occupiers' Liability Act 1957 is statutory law, whereas the principle that the employer must take reasonable care of the health and safety of the employee is common law: a principle laid down by the House of Lords in the case *Wilsons and Clyde Coal Co Ltd v. English* [1937] (*Chapter 5*).

Criminal law relates to actions that can be followed by criminal proceedings in which an accused is prosecuted. Like civil law the sources of criminal law are both statutory and the common law: thus the definition of murder derives from a decision of the courts in the 17th century; whereas the employer's duty to take reasonable care of the employee is not only defined by the common law as part of civil law, but also set out in the Health and Safety at Work Act 1974 and enforced through the criminal courts. Both criminal proceedings and civil proceedings could thus arise from the same set of facts or incidents.

For example, a patient alleged that an unregistered physiotherapist had raped and indecently assaulted her, but the Crown Prosecution Service decided not to prosecute. However, the patient brought a civil action for assault and obtained compensation of over £25000, including an amount representing aggravated damages because the defendant put her through a harrowing ordeal by having to appear in court (*Miles v. Cain* 1988).

Criminal hearings

A prosecution is brought in relation to a charge of a criminal offence and heard in the criminal courts where the standard of proof is beyond reasonable doubt. Summary offences are heard in the Magistrates Court and indictable offences (the more serious offences) in the Crown Court. Many offences are triable either way and the accused can opt for trial by jury. In the Magistrates Court, the magistrates (see below) decide if, on the facts, guilt has been established and, if so, sentence the accused. They also have the power to remit the accused to the Crown Court for sentencing by the Crown Court judge. In the Crown Court, the jury decide if the accused is guilty and, if so, the judge sentences the person convicted.

Criminal negligence

Gross negligence in professional practice may amount to the crime of manslaughter. For example, an anaesthetist failed to realise that during an operation a tube had become disconnected as a result of which the patient

5

died. He was prosecuted in the criminal courts and convicted of manslaughter (*R v. Adomako* 1994) (see *Chapter 4*, p. 36). There would also be liability on his employers in the civil courts for his negligence in causing the death of the patient. The Law Commission (1994) had recommended that the law should be changed to enable it to be made easier for corporations and statutory bodies to be prosecuted for manslaughter. As a result the Corporate Manslaughter and Homicide Act was enacted. Under this the chief executives and chairmen of boards can be found criminally guilty of the offence of corporate manslaughter. (For further details of this Act see *Chapter 4*)

Civil hearings

An action is brought in the civil courts in relation to an alleged civil wrong by a claimant who sues a defendant. The claimant has to satisfy a burden of proving liability on a balance or preponderance of probabilities. There are many kinds of civil action which can be brought: in this book we are principally concerned with the law relating to negligence, breach of the contract of employment and breach of statutory duty.

Public and private law

Another distinction in the classification of laws is that of public and private law. Public law relates to a matter which is a subject of public concern. Thus, the Health and Safety at Work Act is a public law act. Private law relates to matters arising between individuals and/or organisations: thus, a contract of employment places duties upon both employer and employee in relation to health and safety and obeying instructions. An employee could sue the employer for compensation for injuries which have resulted from the employer's failure to take reasonable care of the employee's safety. Public law deals with those areas of law where society intervenes in the actions of individuals. In contrast, private law is concerned with the behaviour of individuals or corporate bodies to each other.

Scotland and Northern Ireland

This book describes the law which applies to England and Wales. For the most part this also applies to Scotland and Northern Ireland, but there are some differences, which are increasing as a result of devolution.

Legal personnel

If a person believes that she has a claim for compensation because of the actions or omissions of health professionals, after possibly seeking advice from the Citizen's Advice Bureau, she would ask a solicitor to take her case. A solicitor is a professionally qualified person (usually possessing a law degree or the Part 1 Common Professional Examinations followed by completion of the Law Society's professional examinations and completion of a set time in supervised practice) who tends to have direct contact with the client. The solicitor may seek the opinion of a barrister (known as counsel) on liability and the amount of compensation. A barrister will usually have a law degree (or have taken the Part I Common Professional Examinations) and must complete the examinations set by the Council for Legal Education. The barrister must be a member of an Inn of Court and complete a term of apprenticeship known as pupillage. Traditionally, the barrister has had the role of conducting the case in court and preparing the documents which are exchanged between the parties in the run up to the court hearing (known as the pleadings). However, recent changes enable either of the professions to represent clients in court, subject only to their having the requisite training.

Procedure in civil courts

Following Lord Woolf's (1996) inquiry, significant changes have been made to civil procedure to simplify and speed up the process. The overriding objective of the civil procedures is to enable the court to deal with cases justly. The emphasis is on attempting to secure a reconciliation of the parties through mediation or alternative dispute resolutions, rather than pursue the case in court. The courts have the responsibility of overseeing cases by what is known as 'case management'.

For personal injury claims under £1000 and other civil claims under £3000, the claim would normally be heard in the Small Claims Court through a process of arbitration. Above these amounts and for claims up to £50000, the claim could be heard in the County Court. Above £50000, the claim would usually be heard in the High Court (divided into three divisions: Chancery, Family and Queen's Bench Division).

Procedure in criminal courts

The magistrates, who are either lay people known as justices of the peace (JPs) and who tend to sit in threes (the bench) or legally qualified persons known as stipendiary magistrates, can only hear charges that relate to offences known as summary offences or offences which can be heard either as summary offences or on indictment (these latter are known as triable either way). Only the Crown Court (with judge and jury) can hear charges of offences which can only be made on indictment (i.e. indictable only offences). Such offences are the most serious, e.g. murder, manslaughter, rape, grievous bodily harm, and other offences against the person, and these can only be heard on indictment in the Crown Court. The magistrates used to have a gate-keeping role in relation to these offences, and oversaw committal proceedings where they decided if there was a case to answer, and if the case should therefore be committed to the Crown Court for the trial to take place. Now a hearing in the Magistrates for arrangements for a plea and case management hearing will take place and the case proceed automatically to the crown court for the trial to take place. In criminal cases, the Crown Prosecution Service (CPS) has the responsibility for preparing the case, including statements, witnesses, etc. for the prosecution in criminal cases.

Accusatorial system

A feature of the legal system in this country is that it consists of one side with the responsibility of proving that the other side is at fault or guilty, or liable, of the wrong or crime alleged. This is known as an accusatorial system and it applies to both civil and criminal proceedings. In criminal cases, the prosecution attempts to show beyond all reasonable doubt that the accused is guilty of the offence with which he is charged. The magistrates, or the jury in the Crown Court, determine whether the prosecution has succeeded in establishing the guilt of the accused, who is presumed innocent until proved guilty.

In civil proceedings, the claimant (originally known as the plaintiff), i.e. the person bringing the action, has to establish on a balance of probability that there is negligence, breach of contract, breach of a statutory duty or whatever civil wrong is alleged. In civil cases (apart from defamation), there is no jury and the judge has the responsibility of determining whether the claimant has succeeded in establishing the civil wrong and, if so, the compensation which should be paid or other remedy. The role of the judge or magistrate is to chair the proceedings, intervening where necessary in the interests of justice, and advising on points of law and procedure.

The accusatorial system contrasts with a system of law which is known as inquisitorial where the judge plays a far more active role in determining the outcome. An example of an inquisitorial system in this country is the Coroner's

Court. Here, the coroner is responsible for deciding which witnesses would be relevant to the answers to the questions which are placed before him by statute (i.e. the identity of the deceased, how, when and where he came to die), and he asks the witnesses questions in court and decides who else can ask questions and what they can ask. As a result of this 'inquisition', he or a jury, if one is used, determine the cause of death. Significant changes to the role and jurisdiction of the coroner are being made following the Shipman Inquiry (Shipman Inquiry Third Report 2003).

Law and ethics

Law is both wider and narrower than the field of ethics. On the one hand, the law covers areas of practice which may not be considered to give rise to any ethical issue, other than the one as to whether the law should be obeyed. For example, to park in a no-parking area would not appear to raise many ethical issues other than the decision to obey or to ignore the law. On the other hand, there are major areas of health care which raise significant ethical questions where there appears to be little law. At any time, of course, a practice which is considered to be contrary to ethical principles can be challenged in court and the judge will make a determination, on the basis of any existing statute law or decided cases, on what the legal position is and thus create a legal precedent.

Situations may arise where a health professional considers the law to be wrong and contrary to her ethical principles. In such a case, she has to decide personally what action to take in full awareness that she could face the effects of the criminal law, civil action, disciplinary procedure by her employer and professional proceedings by the registration body. In certain cases the law itself provides for conscientious objection. Thus, no one can be compelled to participate in a termination of pregnancy unless it is an emergency situation to prevent serious harm to the mother (Abortion Act 1967). Similar provisions apply to activities in relation to human fertilisation and embryology where the Human Fertilisation and Embryology Act 1990 provides a statutory protection clause.

Rules of professional conduct

Professional Associations such as the Society of Radiographers, the Royal College of Nursing, the Royal College of Midwives, the Chartered Society of Physiotherapists and the British Association of Occupational Therapists have issued guidance governing professional practice. Health professional regulation bodies such as the Nursing and Midwifery Council, the Health Professions Council and the General Medical Council have also issued codes of ethics and professional practice. These codes are not in themselves directly enforceable in a court of law, but could be used as evidence in civil or criminal proceedings that their reasonable professional standards of practice have not been followed. An allegation of a breach of the Code of Practice could also be used as a basis for fitness to practise proceedings, for which the ultimate sanction is removal from the Register. Most of the codes of ethics and professional conduct include clauses which relate to health and safety issues.

The new code of professional conduct for nurses and midwives

In June 2008, the Nursing and Midwifery Council (NMC) published its new Standards of conduct, performance and ethics for nurses and midwives (NMC, 2008).

Under the heading Manage Risk, it states:

- You must act without delay if you believe that you, a colleague or anyone else may be putting someone at risk
- You must inform someone in authority if you experience problems that prevent you working within this Code or other nationally agreed standards
- You must report your concerns in writing if problems in the environment of care are putting people at risk

This is a wide-ranging duty and parallels both the statutory duty of the employee under section 7 of the Health and Safety at Work Act 1974 to co-operate with the employer in obeying health and safety regulations and to take care of him/herself and his/her colleagues (*Chapter 2*), and also the duty of the practitioner as an employee under the contract of employment to obey reasonable instructions and to act with reasonable care in carrying out his/her work (*Chapter 5*).

This paragraph recognises the responsibility to raise concerns about health and safety issues.

Failure by the practitioner to observe the Code could result in the practitioner facing fitness to practise proceedings brought by the NMC. The practitioner could also face disciplinary proceedings brought by his/her employer and, in serious cases, could be personally prosecuted in the criminal courts for a health and safety offence.

Other guidance

Many other organisations and public bodies issue guidance for professional conduct and procedures for the provision of health care. The National Health Service Executive and Department of Health issue circulars and executive letters providing advice for health and social services organisations and staff. These do not have the direct force of law, but the Department of Health would expect them to be followed. Directions issued by the Secretary of State under statutory powers are directly enforceable against health service bodies through the default mechanisms provided for in the legislation.

Application of the law of *Scenario 1.1*

Amanda could first see if the staff nurse has any basis for her claim that all patients in A&E departments must be seen by a doctor, by asking her if she is quoting an Act of Parliament of statutory instrument or perhaps directives/regulations from the European Community or is she quoting a ruling by a judge (known as the common law, judge-made law, or case law). The chances are that the staff nurse will have no such authority. In fact, there is no such law in this country whether by statute or common law. Common law does require that every person is entitled to receive a reasonable standard of care when they are treated in hospital, but if this reasonable standard can be delivered by a nurse in the A&E department, there is no requirement that a doctor should also see the patient.

Conclusions

The variety of sources of law and perplexity as to what constitutes a law can be very confusing, but it is helpful for professionals that if they are confronted with a statement that 'the law says...', they seek an explanation as to whether the basis for the assertion is a statute or the decision of a court or is derived from a charter or professional code of practice (which usually do not have the force of law) or, as often may be the case, a pronouncement which is totally incorrect because there is no such law.

References

Davies v. Health and Safety Executive [2002] EWCA Crim 2949, The Times Law Report 27 December 2002

Law Commission Consultative Document on Involuntary manslaughter Paper 135 1994

Lord Woolf (1996) *Final Report Access to Justice*. HMSO, London

Miles v. Cain 25 November 1988 Lexis

Nursing and Midwifery Council (2008) *Standards of Conduct, Performance and Ethics for Nurses and Midwives*. NMC, London

R v. Adomako [1994] 73 ALL ER 79 House of Lords, The Times Law Report July 4 1994

Shipman Inquiry Third Report (2003) Death and Cremation Certification. Available from: www.the-shipman-inquiry.org.uk/reports.asp

Wilsons and Clyde Coal Co Ltd v. English [1937] 3 All ER 628

CHAPTER 2

Statutory provisions on health and safety

> ### Scenario 2.1. Explosion in theatre
>
> Rose is working as a staff nurse in the operating theatre of Roger Park Hospital when there is an explosion. She is severely burnt. Following an inspection by the Health and Safety Inspectorate, the Roger Park NHS Trust is informed that it will be prosecuted. It appears that the cause of the explosion was the result of gases igniting because of an electrical fault in a patient monitor.

Introduction

This chapter considers the basic statutory provisions relating to health and safety and, in particular, it also considers the Provision and use of Work Equipment Regulations 1992 updated 1998. Health and safety laws are a complex mixture of statutory provisions (Acts of Parliament and statutory instruments) and of case law (also known as the common law or judge-made law). Many regulations result from directives from the European Community. Case law both interprets statutory provision and creates new laws where there are gaps in the existing provision (*Chapter 1*). Before the abolition of crown immunity under the National Health Service (Amendment) Act 1986, NHS authorities could not be prosecuted for failures to comply with health and safety laws. Health and safety inspectors visited NHS premises but were unable to issue prohibition and enforcement notices if they found breaches of the Act. Instead, they issued 'crown notices', warning health authorities that if they were not protected by crown immunity, they would be facing a potential prosecution. The immunity was ethically indefensible and since 1986 there have been many prosecutions of health service organisations.

Health and Safety at Work Act 1974: Introduction

The Health and Safety at Work Act creates many statutory duties which are, in the main, of two kinds. Some duties are absolute. For example, Section 2(3) of the Act requires the employer to prepare and, as often as may be appropriate, revise a written statement of his general policy with respect to the health and safety at work of his employees and the organisation, and arrangements for the time being in force for the carrying out of that policy. This is an absolute duty. There are no defences which are available to the employer if there is not in existence a written statement of health and safety policy. The employer could not, for example, argue that it did not have the financial resources or the time to prepare a policy. Similarly, the duty under the Manual Handling Regulations for the employer to carry out a suitable and sufficient assessment of any hazardous manual handling which cannot be avoided is an absolute duty. There can be no defence if the risk assessment has not been carried out (*Chapter 9*).

In contrast, many duties established under the 1974 Act and the regulations drawn up under the Act are duties which must be carried out so far as is reasonably practicable.

Reasonably practicable means that all the circumstances of the situation can be taken into account: the size of the employer's organisation and workforce; the cost of carrying out the duty; the time that it would take. Since such factors are within the knowledge of the employer, section 40 of the 1974 Act enables an employer, when prosecuted for a breach of a reasonably practicable duty under the Act or Regulations, to prove that it took all reasonable practicable means to implement the duty. The employer has to prove that it did this on a balance of probabilities. Clearly, documentation of the risk assessments and action which have been taken would be required to be given in evidence.

Health and Safety at Work Act 1974: Duty of the employer

The basic duty of every employer is set out in Section 2(1) of the Health and Safety at Work Act 1974:

> *It shall be the duty of every employer to ensure,* **so far as is reasonably practicable**, *the health, safety and welfare at work of all his employees.*
>
> [author's emphasis]

Section 2(1) is extremely comprehensive and covers every aspect of the well-being of the employee at work. However, the words in the above quotation which have been put in bold show that the duty is not an absolute one. The employer only has to do what is reasonably practicable. This means that there may be circumstances where an employee is injured at work but a prosecution brought under Section 2(1) against the employer would fail.

The employer may be able to prove on a balance of probabilities that it took all reasonable means to ensure that the employee's health, safety and welfare were safeguarded. To decide what is meant by 'reasonable' would mean looking at the cost, time, value of what the employer has done and any other measures which could reasonably have been taken but were not.

Examples of duties with which the employer must comply

Under Section 2(2) of the 1974 Act examples are given of some of the actions which must be taken by the employer to safeguard the health, safety and welfare of the employer. These detailed duties are shown in *Box 2.1*. These duties cover the safety of equipment and systems of work, use, handling, storage and transport, information, instruction, training and supervision, safe

---

Box 2.1. Section 2(2) Health and Safety at Work Act 1974

Without prejudice to the generality of an employer's duty under the preceding subsection, the matters to which that duty extends include in particular:

(a) The provision and maintenance of plant and systems of work that are, so far as is reasonably practicable, safe and without risks to health

(b) Arrangements for ensuring, so far as is reasonably practicable, safety and absence of risks to health in connection with the use, handling, storage and transport of articles and substances

(c) The provision of such information, instruction, training and supervision as is necessary to ensure, so far as is reasonably practicable, the health and safety at work of his employees

(d) So far as is reasonably practicable as regards any place of work under the employer's control, the maintenance of it in a condition that is safe and without risks to health and the provision and maintenance of means of access to and egress from it that are safe and without such risks

(e) The provision and maintenance of a working environment for his employees that is, so far as is reasonably practicable, safe, without risks to health, and adequate as regards facilities and arrangements for their welfare at work

---

15

premises and a safe working environment. Extensive as these duties are, it must be stressed that these are only examples. They do not detract from the comprehensiveness of the general duty shown in the basic duty on every employer as set out in Section 2(1) of the Health and Safety at Work Act 1974. There would probably have been a breach of some of the specific duties of Section 2(2) in Rose's case in *Scenario 2.1*. In the case of *Pola v. The Crown,* 2009 the Court of Appeal had to rule as to whether a casual Slovakian worker on a building site who worked on a daily basis was an employee of the defendant who was appealing against his conviction of an offence under s.33(1)(a) of the Health and Safety at Work Act 1974 in failing to discharge a duty pursuant to s.2(1) of that Act and of contravention of the Work at Height Regulations. The workman had fallen from a platform and suffered brain damage. The Court of Appeal held that there was sufficient evidence to suggest that an ad hoc contract of employment existed between the man and the employer and therefore dismissed his appeal. It also held that the order of £90000 criminal injury compensation awarded was appropriate.

Employer not liable for deliberate misuse of equipment by an employee

In a Court of Appeal decision (*Horton v. Taplin Contracts Ltd*, 2002) it was held that an employer was not vicariously liable for the deliberate acts of an employee in toppling a scaffolding tower on which the claimant was working, thus causing injuries to the claimant. Also, there was no breach of the Provision and Use of Work Equipment Regulations 1998 (see below) by the employer, since it was not reasonably foreseeable that the other employee would behave as he did. An employer was not liable for breach of statutory duty if the equipment he provided was suitable for use by employees by reference to reasonably foreseeable health and safety hazards and was unsafe only if deliberately misused by an employee.

Health and Safety at Work Act 1974

Duty of employees

The 1974 Act also places very clear legal responsibilities on employees which could also be used as the basis of a prosecution if an employee, including senior management, has failed to comply with the duties. Section 7 which imposes these responsibilities is set out in *Box 2.2*.

> **Box 2.2. Section 7 of the Health and Safety at Work Act 1974**
>
> There is a duty for an employee:
> (a) to take reasonable care for the health and safety of himself and of others who may be affected by his acts or omissions at work
> (b) as regards any duty or requirement imposed on his employer or other person by or under any of the relevant statutory provisions to co-operate with him in so far as is necessary to enable that duty or requirement to be performed or complied with

Duty to the general public

Under Section 3 of the 1974 Act the employers have a general duty of care to persons not in their employment. Employers have a duty to conduct their undertaking in such a way as to ensure, so far as is reasonably practicable, that persons not in their employment who may be affected thereby are not thereby exposed to risks to their health and safety.

This duty would cover patients, visitors and the general public. Like Section 2(1), this duty is not an absolute one, i.e. it is a reasonably practicable one. The burden would be on the employer, if prosecuted, to establish on a balance of probabilities that all reasonable care was taken to protect the general public.

The Court of Appeal has held that, provided the employer has taken all reasonable care in laying down safe systems of work and ensuring that the employees had the necessary skill and instruction and were subject to proper supervision, with safe premises, plant and equipment, the employer was not guilty of an offence under Section 3 of the 1974 Act, if the employee was negligent and caused harm to others (*R v. Nelson Group Services (Maintenance) Ltd* 1998). (The employer might of course be liable in the civil courts for its vicarious liability; this topic will be considered in *Chapter 5*.)

Effect of breach of the general duties

Section 47 states that breach of the general duties (i.e. sections 2–7 and 8) under the Act does not give rise to any form of civil liability. This means that whilst there could be a prosecution in the criminal courts of the employer, an employee or other person, who is a victim and suffered harm as a result of the breach of duty, cannot sue for compensation in the civil courts by reliance on the criminal offence. However, since the general duties are paralleled by duties owed to the employee through the contract of employment or owed to members of the public through the duty of care owed in the law of negligence, an injured person could rely upon these civil actions to claim compensation in the civil courts (*Chapters 5 and 6*). In contrast to the general duties, the breach of many of the regulations may give rise to a claim for compensation in the civil courts.

Regulations

Many regulations have been passed under the Health and Safety at Work Act 1974 defining in greater detail the duties placed upon employer and employee in relation to specific areas of health and safety. Following a European Directive in 1992, six sets of regulations were passed (*Box 2.3*). Many of these regulations have been subsequently amended. The regulations are considered in later chapters of this book. Under the Health and Safety (Miscellaneous Amendments) Regulations 2002 various modifications are made to the regulations relating to, among others, first aid, display screen equipment, manual handling operations, personal protective equipment at work, workplace (health, safety and welfare) provision and use of work equipment, and lifting operations and lifting equipment. The amendments to these regulations can be obtained from the Office of Public Sector Information website, available online at: http://www.opsi.gov.uk/legis.htm

---

Table 2.3. Regulations introduced in January 1993

1. Management of Health and Safety at Work Regulations 1992 (SI (1992) 2051) (revised 1999 SI (1999) No 3242)
2. Provision and Use of Work Equipment Regulations 1992 (SI (1992) 2932) (revised 1998 SI (1998) No 2306)
3. Manual Handling Operations Regulations 1992 (SI (1992) 2793)
4. Workplace (Health, Safety and Welfare Regulations) 1992 (SI (1992) 3004) (amended by SI 1999/2024)
5. Personal Protective Equipment at Work Regulations 1992 (SI (1992) 2966) (amended by SI 1999/3232)
6. Health and Safety (Display Screen Equipment) Regulations 1992 (SI (1992) 2792)

SI = statutory instrument

The manual handling regulations are considered in *Chapter 9*, the provision and use of work equipment regulations are considered below and the management of health and safety at work regulations are discussed in *Chapter 7*.

Provision and Use of Work Equipment Regulations 1992 (PUWER) (revised 1998)

These Regulations were first introduced as part of the six pack set based on an EC Directive in 1992. They were revised in 1998. The regulations cover: the suitability of work equipment, maintenance, inspection, specific risk, information and instructions, training, conformity with community requirements, dangerous parts of machinery, protection against specified hazards, high or very low temperature, controls for starting or making a significant change to operating conditions, (emergency) stop controls, and control systems, isolation from sources of energy, stability, lighting, maintenance operations, markings and warnings. In addition, there are regulations covering mobile work equipment.

The Court of Appeal (*Stark v. Post Office,* 2000) held that Regulation 6(1) of the Provision and Use of Work Equipment Regulations 1992 created an absolute duty. In this case a postman was injured when a part of the front brake of his delivery bicycle broke. (Regulation 6(1) of the 1992 Regulations related to maintenance of equipment, and this is now Regulation 5 of the 1998 Regulations.)

The Court of Session (*Hislop v. Lynx Parcels,* 2003) held in respect of the 1992 Regulations that it was not necessary for a claimant injured as a result of equipment to prove that there was a defect in the equipment for liability to be established under the Regulations. The claimant had been driving a heavy goods vehicle when he observed that a warning light had come on indicating a problem with the radiator. He stopped the vehicle and had gone to inspect the radiator. According to his evidence, the radiator cap had come off. He had not touched the cap. He was struck by scalding water from the radiator, causing burns in various parts of the body. He claimed compensation on the basis of a breach of Regulation 6 of the 1992 PUWER Regulations. The Court held that the obligation of maintenance was an absolute one and applied at all times. It did not matter if the cause of some failure in maintenance remained a mystery. If it was proved that some piece of working equipment had in fact failed, that was sufficient. The Supreme Court held in 2011 (*Baker v Quantum Clothing Group Ltd and others* 2011) in a case relating to the Factories Act 1961 S.29 and which related to events before the Noise at Work Regulations (SI 1989 No 1790) came into force that a workplace could be made unsafe not only because of its physical structure but also as a result of activities carried on in it. Safety had to be judged according to the general knowledge and standards of the times. The onus was on the employee to show that the workplace was unsafe in that basic sense.

House of Lords decision in *Fytche v. Wincanton Logistics plc* (2004)

In the case of *Fytche v. Wincanton Logistics plc* (2004) the House of Lords held that an employer was not liable for an injury caused by a defect in equipment which had no impact on its intended function. In this case, the employer issued his employees with boots with steel toecaps to protect them from impact injuries. However, in a heavy snow storm, a driver, contrary to standard instructions, left his tanker and walked through deep snow. One of his boots leaked and he suffered mild frost bite in his little toe. The House of Lords held that the employers were not in breach of Regulation 7(1) of the Personal Protective Equipment at Work Regulations.

Health and safety legislation to be read together

The guidance of the HSC on the 1998 PUWER regulations emphasises that they cannot be considered in isolation from other health and safety legislation. In particular, they need to be considered with the requirements of the HASAW Act 1974 and the Workplace (Health, Safety and Welfare) Regulations 1992 (revised 1999), the Health and Safety (Display Screen Equipment) Regulations 1992, the Personal Protection Equipment at Work Regulations 1992, and the Management of Health and Safety at Work Regulations 1992 (revised 1999). The latter requires a risk assessment to be carried out, so this requirement is not repeated in PUWER.

Personal Protect Equipment (PPE) at Work Regulations 1992 (as amended)

The Court of Appeal in the case of *Threlfall v. Hull County Council* (2011) ruled that regulations 2 and 4 of the 1992 regulations (SI 1992/2966 as amended by the Health and Safety (Miscellaneous Amendments) Regulations SI 2002/2174) should be interpreted so that the first question should be:

- Does this proposed item of protective equipment prevent or adequately control the identified risk of injury?

The HSE has provided guidance on these regulations under which the employers are responsible for providing, replacing and paying for personal protective equipment. PPE should be used when all other measures are inadequate to control exposure. It protects only the wearer, while being worn. If it fails, PPE offers no protection at all. Types of PPE include respirators, protective gloves, protective clothing, protective footwear, and eye protection The HSE suggests that when deciding about PPE the employer should ask the supplier, the trade association or the manufacturer the following questions:

- Is it suitable for the conditions of the job?
- Does it offer the right level of protection?
- What sort of training or maintenance is required?
- How do I know when it needs replacing?

It is important that employees know why they need PPE and are trained to use it correctly. Otherwise it is unlikely to protect as required.

- Does it fit correctly?
- How does the wearer feel?
- Is it comfortable?
- Are all items of PPE compatible?
- Does PPE interfere with the job being done?
- Does PPE introduce another health risk, e.g. overheating, entanglement with machinery?
- If PPE needs maintenance or cleaning, how is it done?

When employees find PPE comfortable they are far more likely to wear it.

The HSE has published *A Short Guide to the Personal Protective Equipment at Work Regulations* (HSE 1992).

Manslaughter

Individuals who are guilty of breaches of health and safety laws and are grossly negligent in carrying out their duties can face manslaughter charges. In November 2002, it was reported that a fairground safety inspector was jailed for 18 months for failing to spot lethal defects in a ride which led to the deaths of two people (*The Times* 2002). The Corporate Manslaughter and Homicide Act 2007 which introduced a criminal offence by an organisation where gross negligence by senior management causes a death is considered in *Chapter 4*.

Application of the law to *Scenario 2.1*

What is Rose's position? Could she obtain compensation by relying upon breach of these general duties under the Health and Safety at Work Act 1974? Unfortunately, as a consequence of section 47 of the 1974 Act, an employee cannot rely upon breach of the general duties as the basis of an action in the civil courts. However, if the employee could prove that there have been failings by the employer in breach of the contract of employment or in breach of regulations which enable a civil action to be brought, this could be used as the basis of a claim for compensation. In addition, the employer is vicariously liable for any negligence of an employee which causes harm. These topics will be considered in *Chapters 4 and 5*.

References

Baker v. Quantum Clothing Group Ltd and others (2011) The Times Law Report 14 April 2011

Fytche v. Wincanton Logistics plc (2004) The Times Law Report 2 July 2004

Hislop v. Lynx Parcels (2003) Times Law Report 17 April 2003

Horton v. Taplin Contracts Ltd (2002) The Times Law Report 25 November

HSE (1992) *A Short Guide to the Personal Protective Equipment at Work Regulations.* HSE, London

Pola v. The Crown (Health and Safety Executive) [2009] EWCA Crim 655

R v. Nelson Group Services (Maintenance) Ltd (1998) The Times Law Report 17 September 1998 Court of Appeal

Stark v. Post Office (2000) The Times Law Report 29 March 2000

The Times (2002) Adam Fresco Safety Inspector jailed over fair deaths. *The Times* 28 November

Threlfall v. Hull County Council (2011) The Times Law Report 4 March

CHAPTER 3

The role and power of safety representatives and committees

> **Scenario 3.1. Chance to be a safety representative**
>
> Doreen, a radiographer, who had been a union member for many years and more recently had become a union officer in her local branch, was asked by the union if she would like to take on the role of being a health and safety representative. She was hesitant to accept as she was not sure what would be involved.

Introduction

This chapter discusses the role and powers of safety representatives and the establishment of safety committees which were set up under the Health and Safety at Work Act 1974. The philosophy within the Robens Report (Robens Committee 1972), which preceded the Health and Safety at Work Act 1974, was that good standards in health and safety within the workplace should result from co-operation between employer and employee. The employees should ensure that risks and hazards of which they were aware were made known to the employer. The employer would then wish to fulfil its duty of taking the necessary measures to ensure that accidents, ill health and industrial diseases were prevented. If this communication and co-operation worked successfully, there would be no need for the more draconian measure of notices and prosecution by health and safety inspectors. The Health and Safety at Work Act 1974 made provision for the appointment of health and safety representatives and the establishment of health and safety committees. Regulations were made in 1977 and these will be considered in the light of the situation in *Scenario 3.1*.

Safety representatives

The Safety Representatives and Safety Committee Regulations (SRSCR) 1977 (SI 1977, No. 500) laid down the basis of the powers and duties of safety representatives. Safety representatives are appointed by a recognised trade union from among the employees. The employer is notified of the name of the appointed person. As set out in section 2(4) of the 1974 Act, the safety representative has the task of representing the employees in consultations with the employers and other duties set out in the regulations. The HSE (2008) has provided guidance for employers and workers on the regulations and the functions of the safety representatives. The HSE has published the 'Brown Book' (Safety Representatives and Safety Committees Regulations 1977, Approved Code of Practice and Guidance) for training purposes for the Trade Union Congress.

Under section 2(6) of the Health and Safety at Work Act 1974, the employers have a duty to consult any safety representatives with a view to the making and maintenance of arrangements that will enable them, and their employees, to co-operate effectively in promoting and developing measures to ensure the health and safety at work of the employees and in checking the effectiveness of such measures. The functions of the safety representatives can be seen in *Box 3.1*.

The 1974 Act specifically states that the functions (*Box 3.1*) are not to be seen as imposing any duty on the safety representative. This means that failure by safety representatives to fulfil these functions could not render them liable to

---

Box 3.1. Functions of health and safety representatives

- To investigate potential hazards and dangerous occurrences in the workplace
- To investigate complaints by any employee they represent relating to that employee's health, safety or welfare at work
- To make representations to the employer on matters arising out of the above
- To make representations to the employer on general matters affecting the health, safety or welfare of the employees
- To carry out inspections
- To present the employees in consultations with inspectors of the health and safety inspectorate or any other enforcing authority
- To receive information from inspectors
- To attend meetings of safety committees where they attend in their capacity as safety representatives

Source: Safety Representative and Safety Committee Regulations 1977
(SI 1977, No. 500)

---

prosecution or civil liability. Of course, as an employee, safety representatives remain liable under the statutory duty under section 7 of the Health and Safety at Work Act 1974 to co-operate with the employer and to take reasonable care of the health and safety of both themselves and their colleagues (*Chapter 2*).

Where employees are not represented under the Safety Representatives and Safety Committees Regulations 1977, the Health and Safety (Consultation with Employees) Regulations 1996 will apply (*see below*). Thus the 1996 Regulations would apply where there is no recognised trade union, or where there is a recognised trade union but no safety representative has been appointed.

The HSE has provided many publications including: *Consulting Employees on Health and Safety: A brief guide to the law (INDG232); Involving Your Workforce in Health and Safety: Good practice for workplaces (HSG263)* and *Consulting Your Workforce on Health and Safety. Approved Code of Practice and Guidance* (L146) (HSE 2008). The booklet on involving your workforce in health and safety gives practical advice to employers on the following topics:

- Getting started: Prepare
- Getting organised: Plan
- Getting it done: Consult and involve
- Getting it right: Keep improving

It contains many useful checklists and is written in an accessible way. It can be downloaded from the HSE website, as can all HSE publications.

Paid time off work

The employer is obliged to permit the safety representative to take such time off with pay during the employee's working hours as shall be necessary for the purposes of performing these functions, and undergoing such training in aspects of those functions as may be reasonable in all the circumstances. If an employer fails to give paid time off work to the safety representative, then the latter can make an application to an employment tribunal (Regulation 11, SRSCR).

Specific powers are given under paragraphs 5 and 6 of the SRSCR in relation to the inspection of the workplace, and inspections following notifiable accidents, occurrences and diseases. The employer is required to provide such facilities and assistance as the safety representative may reasonably require (including facilities for independent investigation by them and private discussion with employees) for the purpose of carrying out an investigation. The regulations do not prevent the employer or its representative being present during the inspection.

The employer, on receipt of a request in writing, is also required under paragraph 7 of the Regulations to provide the safety representative with information which the employer is obliged to keep under the Health and Safety at Work Act 1974 and other statutory provisions. Exceptions to this requirement include any disclosure which:

- would be contrary to the interests of national security,
- would identify an individual unless he/she has consented, or
- would cause substantial injury to the employer's undertaking, or
- includes any information obtained by the employer for the purpose of bringing, prosecuting or defending any legal proceedings.

Health and safety committees

Under section 2(7) of the Health and Safety at Work Act 1974 the employer has the duty, if requested by the safety representative, to establish a safety committee which has the function of keeping under review the measures taken to ensure the health and safety at work of its employees and such other functions as may be prescribed. Regulation 9 of SRSCR sets out how employers are to fulfil their duty to establish a safety committee when requested. They are required to consult with the safety representative making the request, and with representatives of any recognised trade unions. They must then post a notice stating the composition of the committee and the workplace covered and the committee shall be established not later than three months after the request is made. The HSE has provided guidance entitled *Health and Safety Committees: Setting them up and making them work* (HSE 2010).

Health and Safety (Consultation with Employees) Regulations 1996

As a result of an EC Directive (Council Directive 89/391/EEC, OJ. No L183, 29.6.89, p1), the Health and Safety (Consultation with Employees) Regulations 1996 (SI 1996, No 1513) were passed which applied to those workplaces which are not covered by SRSCR. All employers are required to consult with workers or their representatives on matters relating to employees' health and safety, whether or not there are recognised trade unions in the workplace. Similar rights in relation to reasonable paid time off for carrying out functions and having training are given, together with the duty on the employer to make certain information available. Similarly, the Regulations do not create any civil liability in respect of any breach of duties by the representatives.

The specified functions of representatives under the 1996 Regulations are to make representations to the employer on potential hazards and dangerous occurrences at the workplace and on general matters affecting health and safety at work, and to represent the group of employees they represent in consultations at the workplace with health and safety inspectors. Representatives who are dismissed or suffer a detriment as a result of undertaking these health and safety functions are entitled to obtain redress from the employment tribunal.

Management of Health and Safety at Work Regulations 1999

The Management of Health and Safety at Work Regulations (SI 1999, No 3242) originally drawn up in 1992 (SI 1992, No. 2051) and modified in 1999 contain important provisions in relation to the giving of information to employees. Regulation 10 requires every employer to provide his employees with comprehensible and relevant information on the risks to their health and safety identified by an assessment, the preventive and protective measures, the procedures for dealing with serious and imminent dangers and the identity of the persons who are to implement these procedures. These regulations are considered further in *Chapter 7* on risk management.

Application of the law to *Scenario 3.1*

Doreen will find that her union will have a considerable amount of printed information about the role of the safety representative and her powers and rights. She will be able to claim paid time off to carry out her duties and also for training in her new role. If possible, she could talk to her predecessor to find out more information and any particular problems in her specific workplace. Clearly, her new role would be facilitated by a proactive and supportive management. There will be considerable time demands which she will need to take into account in securing a balance between her present post and how she could take on new union responsibilities. She is also likely to find that the more successful she is in resolving the health and safety worries of her colleagues, the more concerns her colleagues are likely to bring to her.

Conclusion

It was perhaps unrealistic for the Robens Report (1972) to consider that health and safety standards could be left to co-operation between employers and employees and prosecutions would have a minimum role to play. As long as health and safety duties are in the main not absolute, but only 'reasonably practicable', then employers confronted by the demands of the representatives at health and safety committees could argue that they had not the resources to make the necessary improvements. In addition, they could state that the costs of improving health and safety standards outweighed the benefits to be achieved by that expenditure. With such responses to legitimate demands by health and safety representatives it is little wonder that health and safety committees were seen merely as a talking shop and no action could be expected from them. There is, however, still a place for the role of the safety representative, and also, where management is anxious to take risk assessment and management procedures seriously, for the existence of health and safety committees. The National Patient Safety Agency (*Chapter 13*) may have encouraged effective working of both health and safety representatives and health and safety committees as part of its overall objective of learning from the lessons across the NHS and implementing the necessary action.

References

Robens Committee (1972) *Robens Committee Report on Safety and Health at Work.* Cmnd 5034. HMSO, London

HSE (2008) *Consulting Your Workforce on Health and Safety. Safety Representatives and Safety Committees Regulations 1977 (as amended) and Health and Safety (Consultation with Employees) Regulations 1996 (as amended). Approved Code of Practice and guidance L146.* HSE Books, London

HSE (2008) *Consulting Employees on Health and Safety: A brief guide to the law INDG232(rev1).* HSE Books, London

HSE (2008) *Involving Your Workforce in Health and Safety: Good practice for all workplaces HSG263.* HSE Books, London

HSE (2010) *Health and Safety Committees: Setting them up and making them work.* HSE Books, London

CHAPTER 4

Enforcement of statutory duties for health and safety at work

---

Scenario 4.1: A scalding

Bert, aged 85 years, suffered from Alzheimer's disease and had been in hospital for several weeks. One day, a nursing auxiliary filled the bath with water while another fetched him from the ward and brought him to the bathroom in a wheelchair. He was placed in the hoist and lowered into the bath. He screamed out in agony and was severely scalded. Chris, the staff nurse on duty, was concerned that she could be prosecuted. What is the law?

Introduction

Under the Health and Safety at Work Act 1974 some new institutions responsible for ensuring the implementation of health and safety laws across the country were established. These included the Health and Safety Commission (HSC), the Health and Safety Executive (HSE) and the Health and Safety Inspectorate. Subsequently on 1 April 2008 the Health and Safety Commission was merged into the Health and Safety Executive. Information can be obtained from its website (www.hse. gov.uk) where it was stated:

> *To improve governance arrangements, the Health and Safety Commission and the current three person Health and Safety Executive agreed to merge into a new unitary body, bringing together their powers and functions, and retaining the name Health and Safety Executive. In doing so, they were committed to maintaining the current legal position whereby only duly authorised officials make individual enforcement decisions. A new authorisation instrument was drawn up. (The Legislative Reform (Health and Safety Executive) Order 2008 (S.I.2008/960))*

Health and Safety Executive (HSE)

The HSE is responsible to the Secretary of State for the Environment, Transport and the Regions and to other Secretaries of State for the administration of the Health and Safety at Work Act 1974. The functions of the HSE are set out in *Box 4.1*.

Box 4.1. Functions of the Health and Safety Executive

- To secure the health, safety and welfare of persons at work
- To protect the public generally against risks to health or safety arising out of work activities and to control the keeping and use of explosives, highly flammable and other dangerous substances
- To conduct and sponsor research, promote training and provide an information and advisory service
- To review the adequacy of health and safety legislation and submit to the Government proposals for new and revised regulations and approved codes of practice

---

The statutory functions of the HSE include making adequate arrangements for enforcement of the statutory provisions of the 1974 Act (*Chapter 2*). It also has the power to appoint inspectors. The HSE maintains an employment medical advisory service (EMAS) which gives advice and information concerning the safeguarding and improvement of health of people at work. The HSE also supports police investigations into possible work-related manslaughter offences. In 2000/2001, the police referred 22 cases of work-related death in sectors, where the HSE was the enforcement authority, to the Crown Prosecution Service to consider possible manslaughter charges (see below).

Health and Safety Inspectorate

Appointed by the HSE, the Health and Safety Inspectorate has the statutory powers under section 20 of the Health and Safety at Work Act 1974 to enforce health and safety laws. Its powers are summarised in *Box 4.2*. The HSE inspects most workplaces, including hospitals. Certain places, including offices, hotels, catering and residential accommodation, are inspected by local authority environment officers.

Box 4.2. Powers of Health and Safety Inspectors
S.20 of Health and Safety of Work Act 1974

(1) An inspector may, for the purpose of carrying into effect any of the relevant statutory provisions within the field of responsibility of the enforcing authority which appointed him, exercise the powers set out in subsection (2) below.

(2) The powers of an inspector referred to in the preceding subsection are the following, namely:

(a) at any reasonable time enter any premises which he has reason to believe it is necessary for him to enter for the purpose mentioned in subsection (1) above;

(b) to take with him a constable if he has reasonable cause to apprehend any serious obstruction in the execution of his duty;

(c) on entering any premises by virtue of paragraph (a) above to take with him:

  (i) any other person duly authorised by his (the inspector's) enforcing authority; and

  (ii) any equipment or materials required for any purpose for which the power of entry is being exercised;

(d) to make such examination and investigation as may in any circumstances be necessary for the purpose mentioned in subsection (1) above;

(e) direct that those premises or any part of them, or anything therein, shall be left undisturbed (whether generally or in particular respects) for so long as is reasonably necessary for the purpose of any examination or investigation under paragraph (d) above;

(f) to take such measurements and photographs and make such recordings as he considers necessary for the purpose of any examination or investigation under paragraph (d) above;

(g) to take samples of any articles or substances;

(h) in the case of any article or substance found in any premises cause it to be dismantled or subjected to any process or test;

(i) in the case of any such article or substance as is mentioned in the preceding paragraph, to take possession of it and detain it for so long as is

Box 4.2 cont/

Box 4.2 cont/

necessary for all or any of the following purposes, namely:
(i) to examine it and do to it anything which he has power to do under that paragraph;
(ii) to ensure that it is not tampered with before his examination of it is completed;
(iii) to ensure that it is available for use as evidence in any proceedings for an offence under any of the relevant statutory provisions or any proceedings relating to a notice under section 21 or 22;
(j) if he is conducting an examination or investigation under (d) to require any person ... to answer any questions as the inspector thinks fit and to sign a declaration of the truth of his answers;
(k) to require production of, inspect and take copies of any entry in any books or documents;
(l) to require any person to afford himself such facilities and assistance within that person's control or responsibilities as are necessary for him to exercise his powers;
(m) any other power which is necessary for the purpose of exercising any of the above powers.

The HSE has produced a leaflet, *What to Expect When a Health and Safety Inspector Calls* (HSE, 1998). This leaflet provides guidance on the powers of the inspectors and the enforcement actions that they may take if they are aware of breaches of the law. The enforcement actions include:

- Informal: advice to the employer on compliance.
- Improvement notice: a formal notice to advise the employer on how to comply with the law within a period specified in the notice.
- Prohibition notice: if an activity could cause serious personal injury, this notice can be issued to prohibit the activity until remedial action has been taken.
- Prosecution: failure to comply with a prohibition or improvement notice. Prosecution can also follow other breaches of health and safety laws.

The HSE provided guidance in 2010 for other people to accompany enforcement officers on site. Under section 20(2)(c)(i) of the Health and Safety at Work etc Act 1974, an inspector may take another person with them on an inspection, e.g. a person with expert knowledge of the type of workplace being visited. Prior authorisation by the Enforcing Authority should be arranged for the person concerned, otherwise they will not have any right of entry to the premises. This could cause delays during emergency situations. The Guidance includes a form which could be used to cover the visit.

The HSE publishes an annual report on health and safety offences and penalties. The report for April 2000–March 2001 shows that in 2000–2001 there were 40 visits to NHS trusts or private hospitals, some of which were follow-up visits to NHS trusts which had already been the subject of a management inspection. The issues which were used as key performance indicators for these inspections are shown in *Box 4.3*.There were 43 improvement notices issued: 12 on general health and safety management, 11 on control of substances hazardous to health (COSHH), four on manual handling, four on violence to staff and four on hot water management. There were 21 prosecutions, over half of which were related to inadequate control of hot water/hot surfaces. In the annual report for 2009–2010 the incidence rate for fatal and major injuries per 100 000 employees had fallen from 117.3 in 1999–2000 to 105.6 in 2008–2009. Separate figures are not given for the NHS. In 2000–2002 there were 1.76 days lost per worker from work-related injury or ill-health; the corresponding figure for 2008–2009 is 1.24.

Box 4.3. Key performance indicators for inspections

- Management of manual handling
- Management of control of substances hazardous to health (COSHH), control of infection, exposure to glutaraldehyde and latex
- Managing the risks from workplace violence
- Hot water management – the control of risks from scalding
- *Legionella spp.*

Accountability of the HSE

An action was brought against a Health and Safety Inspector on the grounds that negligent advice had been given to local authorities which had refused to permit a crane to be used for bungee jumping (*Harris v. Evans and another* 1998). The claimant had suffered severe economic loss as a result of the negligent advice.

The Court of Appeal held that no duty of care was owed by the inspector to the proprietor of any business affected by their notices. The purpose of the 1974 Act was to protect the public and extensive powers were available to an inspector for that purpose. To impose a duty of care would be likely to engender untoward cautiousness, and the temptation to postpone making a decision until further inquiries had been made would be seriously detrimental to the proper discharge by enforcing authorities of their responsibilities.

HSE strategy: Health and safety of Great Britain

The HSE published its strategy for the health and safety of GB in 2009. As part of the strategy the Health and Safety Pledge Forum was launched on 24 February 2010. The Strategy encouraged organisations to show their commitment to workplace health and safety by signing the HSE Safety Pledge.

HSE (2009) stated that it was

...keen for those who have signed the Pledge to share ideas for improving health and safety with each other or to work with HSE on collaborative ventures in risk management. The Pledge Forum helps this process by allowing pledge signers to share ideas and best practice and ask questions. It also contains a wealth of information on a range of topics including: worker protection; absence management; saving recruitment and insurance costs; improving productivity; reputation management; and case studies for both small/medium sized businesses and large businesses.

Prosecutions brought by the HSE

In *Chapter 2* the case of *Pola v. The Crown (Health and Safety Executive)* [2009] is considered in which the employer argued unsuccessfully that the injured worker was not employed by him and that the compensation awarded should be reduced.

BUPA Care Homes (BNH) Ltd was fined £150000 following a prosecution by the HSE after a pensioner died at a nursing home in Birmingham. (HSE Release No:WM329/11)

Seventy-four-year-old Brigid O'Callaghan, known as Vera, died after being strangled by a lap belt when she was left strapped in a wheelchair overnight. Birmingham Crown Court heard that staff at the company's Amberley Court Nursing Home, on Edgbaston Road, Edgbaston, did not properly check on Mrs O'Callaghan on the night of 27 October 2005, leaving her in a wheelchair in her room rather than helping her to bed. She was discovered dead the next morning by a member of staff having slipped from the seat of the wheelchair to the floor, with the lap belt strap around her neck. An HSE investigation into safety standards at the home following Mrs O'Callaghan's death found more than 15 failings in her treatment. The court heard that the home had failed to carry out a proper risk assessment and care plan for Mrs O'Callaghan's stay, did not communicate her needs to staff, failed to ensure she could call for help and did not monitor whether night time checks were carried out. HSE inspectors also identified more than 10 further potential hazards that put residents at risk, ranging from a cluttered corridor to dirty conditions. These included the absence of window restraints; excessive water temperature in two bathrooms; failure to secure a laundry room; tripping hazards and charging a battery in a corridor; storing lifting slings over a handrail; inappropriate treatment of waste items and laundry; dirty conditions of a shower and toilet; inappropriate storage of items in bathrooms; failure to secure a housekeeping room; a cluttered corridor; insufficient resources for an adequate maintenance programme; insufficient monitoring of the management of the home; and lack of staff training. BUPA Care Homes pleaded guilty to two breaches of Section 3(1) of the Health and Safety at Work Act 1974. The first charge focused on the issues most closely connected to Mrs O'Callaghan's death and the second on the potential hazards for the other residents. The company was fined £150000 in total and ordered to pay £150000 in costs. HSE inspector Sarah Palfreyman said:

Mrs O'Callaghan's death was a preventable tragedy caused by a shocking case of mismanagement. The managers of this, and indeed all care homes, have a duty of care for their residents. At the very least they should be making sure that residents are comfortable and safe at night, not left in a wheelchair. There were some awful conditions for the elderly residents to live in and hazards that could easily have caused them serious injury. The home's managers were not given appropriate monitoring or supervision and as a result the staff were not being properly trained or monitored. Working in a care home is a specialised job and it's vital that all employees have the correct training in place, which in this instance, they did not.

Prosecution under Section 3(1) of HASAW 1974

An elderly woman died of her injuries after being thrown from a wheelchair while in an Age Concern Westminster minibus. Olive Sarti, 88, was taken to hospital with a head injury and a broken neck after the incident on 20 September

2006. The HSE prosecuted Age Concern Westminster after an investigation that found the minibus driver had performed an emergency stop which resulted in Ms Sarti being hurled from her wheelchair. The elderly lady was taken to hospital with a broken neck and head injuries. She died two months later on 11 November 2006. The employees had not secured Ms Sarti in her wheelchair, and the workers had not been given adequate training by the charity to ensure wheelchair users were safe while travelling. Age Concern Westminster of Praed Street, Westminster, London was found guilty of breaching Section 3(1) of the Health and Safety at Work etc Act 1974. It was fined £10000 and ordered to pay costs of £5000.

HSE Inspector Michael La Rose said:

'This fatal incident was foreseeable. There was MHRA guidance easily available to Age Concern Westminster on how to transport wheelchair users safely. This organisation fell well below expected standards and Olive Sarti's death could have been avoided if Age Concern Westminster workers had received adequate training. The seatbelt laws have long been established in British law. Age Concern was aware that people transported in wheelchairs should have these effectively secured and the wheelchair user should have an adequate seatbelt.

Manslaughter charges

An example of a manslaughter charge was the decision to prosecute a local authority for manslaughter over the deaths of seven people from Legionnaire's disease (Ford 2004). The Crown Prosecution Service decided not only to press charges against Barrow Borough Council but also against one of its employees, a design manager, for gross negligence amounting to manslaughter. It was alleged by the CPS that the disease was caused by a 30-year-old air conditioning unit at the council-operated Forum 28 arts complex in August 2002. After the outbreak it was discovered that the maintenance contract to clean the unit where the bacteria grew had been terminated. Cleaning was then done by the Council. Subsequently the Corporate Manslaughter and Corporate Homicide Act 2007 was brought into force (see below).

Thames Trains was fined £2 million following the Paddington rail crash in which 31 people were killed (Smith 2004). It had pleaded guilty in December 2003 at Bow Street magistrates court to two charges under Health and Safety legislation that it had failed to ensure as far as was reasonably practicable the health and safety of its employees and passengers under the 1974 Act.

An individual health professional could be convicted of manslaughter if he or she acted in such a grossly negligent way that the death of a patient is caused. To convict, the jury must be satisfied beyond reasonable doubt, that there was gross negligence and that this caused the death of the victim. In the leading case of *R v. Adomako,* where a patient had died on the operating table when a tube bringing gases to the patient had become disconnected, the anaesthetist claimed that, whilst he may have been negligent, he was not guilty of a criminal offence. However the House of Lords laid down the following principles:

1. The ordinary principles of the law of negligence should be applied to ascertain whether or not the defendant had been in breach of a duty of care towards the victim who had died.
2. If such a breach of duty was established, the next question was whether that breach caused the death of the victim.
3. If so, the jury had to go on to consider whether that breach of duty should be characterised as gross negligence and therefore as a crime. That would depend on the seriousness of the breach of duty committed by the defendant in all the circumstances in which the defendant was placed when it occurred.
4. The jury would have to consider whether the extent to which the defendant's conduct departed from the proper standard of care incumbent upon him, involving as it must have done a risk of death to the patient, was such that it should be judged criminal.
5. The judge was required to give the jury a direction on the meaning of gross negligence as had been given in the present case by the Court of Appeal.
6. The jury might properly find gross negligence on proof of:
   (a) indifference to an obvious risk of injury to health, or of
   (b) actual foresight of the risk coupled either
      (i) with a determination nevertheless to run it or
      (ii) with an intention to avoid it but involving such a high degree of negligence in the attempted avoidance as the jury considered justified conviction, or
   (c) of inattention or failure to advert to a serious risk going beyond mere inadvertence in respect of an obvious and important matter which the defendant's duty demanded he should address.

(Lettering and numbering are the author's)

Corporate Manslaughter and Corporate Homicide Act 2007

The Corporate Manslaughter and Corporate Homicide Act was enacted in 2007. It does the following:

- It abolishes the common law offence of corporate manslaughter by gross negligence.
- It creates statutory offences which can be committed by a specified organisation.
- Prosecution can be brought if the activities of the organisation are managed or organised in a way which causes a person's death, and amounts to a gross breach of a relevant duty of care owed by the organisation to the deceased.
- An organisation is guilty of an offence under this section only if the way in which its activities are managed or organised by its senior management is a substantial element in the breach of the duty of care.
- The organisations specified include 'corporations' and also the Department of Health.
- The duty of care includes duties to a detained patient, but excludes any duty of care owed by a public authority in respect of a decision as to matters of public policy (including in particular the allocation of public resources or the weighing of competing public interests).
- Duty of care also excludes emergency responses carried out by an NHS body or ambulance service.

The first case of a prosecution under the Corporate Manslaughter and Corporate Homicide Act was of Cotswold Geotechnical Holdings which was accused of gross negligence leading to the death of a geologist who died whilst taking soil samples when the pit he was working in collapsed on him. Peter Eaton, a director, became ill and the trial was adjourned to be preceded by a pre-trial assessment of Eaton's mental condition (*The Times* 2009). Subsequently the charges against Eaton were stayed, but the charges against the Company under the Corporate Manslaughter and Homicide Act and under the Health and Safety at Work Act proceeded. The company was fined £385000. No one was in the dock for the three week trial and the business denied corporate manslaughter (*The Times* 2011).

Guidelines for sentencing for corporate manslaughter were published by the Sentencing Guidelines Council in February 2010.

The Health and Safety (Offences) Act 2008

The Health and Safety (Offences) Act 2008 came into force on 16 January 2009. Under the provisions of the Act, offenders who break the law are subjected to higher fines and longer sentences. The Act makes imprisonment an option for more health and safety offences in both the lower and higher courts.

It also allows certain offences which at one time could only be tried in lower courts, to be tried in the higher courts. The main change that the Act has brought is to raise the maximum fine which may be imposed in the lower courts to £20000 for most health and safety offences.

Application of the law to the situation in *Scenario 4.1*

The injuries to Bert must be reported to the HSE, who would probably visit the hospital and undertake an investigation into the accident (it should be noted that temperature control is one of the HSE's key performance indicators; see *Box 4.3*).

It is highly probable that the inspectors will find that there were serious failures in relation to temperature controls and that there was a lack of a safe system of work. There is likely to be a prosecution of the NHS trust which has failed to comply with health and safety duties, in particular section 3 (which places a duty on the employer to the wider public (see *Chapter 2*), and the general duty of an employer to conduct its undertaking in such a way as to ensure, so far as is reasonably practicable, that persons not in his/her employment who may be affected are not thereby exposed to risks to their health and safety (*Chapter 2*). If Bert were to die from his injuries, the HSE would co-operate with the police in passing information with a view to a prosecution for manslaughter by the Crown Prosecution Service. The Inspectorate would also consider carefully the specific responsibilities on the ward to ensure that patients were safe. This would include ascertaining who had responsibility for training the nursing auxiliaries when bathing patients. If it were to be established that specific employees were in breach of section 7 of the Health and Safety at Work Act 1974 then an individual employee could be prosecuted (section 7 requires all employees to take reasonable care of themselves and others and to co-operate with employers in implementing health and safety statutory responsibilities (see *Chapter 2*). It may well be, therefore, that Chris will be interviewed by the health and safety inspectors and will have to satisfy them that she was not at fault in causing the scalding of the patient. She would have to answer questions about her health and safety responsibilities and the scalding of the patient and she may be required to provide a statement. She should seek assistance from a senior manager or solicitor to the trust in making this statement.

Conclusion

The abolition of crown immunity enjoyed by health authorities has fundamentally changed the relationship of the HSE and inspectors with the NHS. Instead of powerless warnings, the inspectorate has the same powers of enforcement against health service employers which it has against non-NHS employers. The Health and Safety at Work (Offences) Act 2008 made provision for the prosecution and punishment of offences which are treated as offences under the Health and Safety at Work Act 1974 or the Employers' Liability (Compulsory Insurance) Act 1969 and provides a new schedule of punishments. Higher fines and longer sentences may have a deterrent effect on health and safety offending and the Corporate Manslaughter and Homicide Act may also assist in raising health and safety standards.

We have concentrated in this chapter on the main enforcement bodies of Health and Safety legislation but the Better Regulation Task Force, set up by the Government has pointed out that the NHS must satisfy 36 separate regulators. The chairman of the task force, David Arculus, considered that the NHS was the greatest victim of regulatory excess. Lord Young was commissioned by the Prime Minister in 2009 to review Health and Safety laws. His report, which was welcomed by the HSE, is discussed in *Chapter 24*.

References

Ford R (2004) Manslaughter charges over legionella deaths. *The Times*: 11 February

Harris v. Evans and another [1998] 3 All ER 522

HSE (1998) *What to Expect When a Health and Safety Inspector Calls*. HSE, London. Available from: www.hse.gov.uk/ pubns/hsc14.htm

Law Commission (1996) *Report No 237 Legislating the Criminal Code: Involuntary manslaughter*. Stationery Office, London

Pola v. The Crown (Health and Safety Executive) [2009] EWCA Crim 655

R v. Adomako [1994] 73 ALL ER 79 House of Lords, The Times Law Report July 4 1994

Sentencing Guidelines Council (2010) *Corporate Manslaughter and Health and Safety Offences Causing Death: Definitive Guideline* SGC, London

Smith L (2004) Thames Trains fined £2 m over Paddington crash. *The Times*: 6 April

The Times (2009) Manslaughter by negligence case. *The Times:* 24 April

The Times (2011) News item. *The Times*: 18th February

The HSE produces a large number of free and priced publications. A free catalogue and the publications are available by mail order from:

HSE Books, PO Box 1999, Sudbury, Suffolk CO10 6FS. Tel: 01787 881165; Fax: 01787 313995.

For other enquiries telephone the HSE's InfoLine: 0845 345 0055, or write to HSE InfoLine, Caerphilly Business Park, Caerphilly CF83 3GG

HSE website: http://www.hse.gov.uk

CHAPTER 5

Contractual and common law responsibilities

Scenario 5.1. Duty of the employer

Violet was a staff nurse working on a ward at Roger Park Hospital with patients with infectious diseases. She claimed that there was inadequate equipment to ensure safe practices in preventing cross-infection between patients and staff. She then discovered that she had contracted hepatitis B and it seemed likely that she had been infected by a patient. She wishes to obtain compensation.

Introduction

In *Chapter 2* it was noted that breach of the general duties of the Health and Safety at Work Act 1974 could not be used as the basis of a claim for compensation in the civil courts. In the situation in *Chapter 2*, Rose was burnt in an explosion in theatre and could not sue for compensation for her injuries on the basis of breach of the general duties set out in the Health and Safety at Work Act 1974. However, it was pointed out that she may be able to sue for compensation for breach of the employer's contractual duty to take reasonable care of her health and safety. This chapter considers the contractual duties owed by the employer to take reasonable care of the health and safety of the employee and the contractual duties of the employee in relation to health and safety.

The direct duty of the employer to care for the safety of the employee

When a person or organisation agrees to employ another person then a contract of employment comes into existence between them. The terms of this contract are contained in a variety of sources:

- The letter of appointment or agreed by word of mouth at the interview.
- A collection of terms agreed through the process of collective bargaining

(such as the NHS Pay Review Body and the specific terms for the different categories of staff).

- Acts of Parliament and statutory instruments may require employers to recognise certain terms which give rights to employees, e.g. statutory sick pay, maternity benefits.
- Terms implied by law.

Implied terms

As a result of decisions by the courts some of the terms added to a contract of employment are implied by the common law. These implied terms place duties upon both employer and employee. Under these duties implied into the contract of employment, the employer has an obligation to safeguard the health and safety of the employee. This implied term has been interpreted as requiring the employer to:

- employ competent staff,
- set up a safe system of work,
- maintain safe premises, equipment and plant.

If the employer has failed to take such reasonable care for the health and safety of the employee, then the employee may have a claim for breach of contract by the employer and the employee would be able to obtain compensation in the civil courts. This principle was laid down by the House of Lords in 1937 (*Wilsons and Clyde Coal Co Ltd v. English* 1937).

Effect of failures by the employer

Failure by the employer to take reasonable care of the health, safety or welfare of the employee could result in the following actions by the employee:

- Action for breach of contract of employment.
- Action for negligence, where the employee has suffered harm; the employee could also use as evidence breach of specific health and safety regulations.
- Application in the employment tribunal for constructive dismissal, if it can be shown that the employer is in fundamental breach of the contract of employment. (The concept of constructive dismissal enables an employee who is faced with fundamental failures by the employer in fulfilling

contractual conditions to argue that the contract has been ended by reason of the conduct of the employer. In law this ending of the contract is seen as a dismissal.)

Implied duties placed upon the employee

Implied terms in the contract of employment require the employee:

*   To obey the reasonable instructions of the employer.
*   To take reasonable care and skill in carrying out the work.

Failure by the employee to comply with these terms could lead to the employer taking disciplinary action against the employee, and ultimately the dismissal of the employee. The employee may have the right of applying to an employment tribunal for unfair dismissal.

Actual or constructive knowledge of risk

The Court of Appeal has held that it was a matter of fact in each case whether an employer had constructive knowledge of a serious risk, so as to trigger its duty of care towards employees (*Doherty and others v. Rugby Joinery (UK) Ltd* 2004). In the case itself the employees suffered from vibration-induced white finger and the judge held that it was agreed that the employer did not have actual knowledge of this risk nor at that time was it reasonable to expect the employer to have constructive knowledge of the risk.

A health service example: *Fraser v. Winchester Health Authority*

A girl aged 21 was employed as a resident support worker at a home for mentally and physically disabled residents run by Winchester Health Authority. She was sent on a week's camping holiday with a patient without supervision of assistance. She had no training or instruction in the use of camping equipment. She suffered burns to her face and hands when, needing to cook an evening meal for the patient, she changed the cylinder on a gas cooker at the entrance to the tent and near to a lit candle. There was an explosion and the tent caught fire. The Court of Appeal held that a young, inexperienced support worker with the heavy responsibility for looking after her patient was provided with the bare minimum of equipment and no instruction. To compound its failure, the defendant health authority had sent the support worker out with candles and matches which could only suggest to her that they might be used in the tent to provide light. The claimant however was one third responsible because she fully recognised the risk in what she did, so she was held to be a third contributorily negligent (see below). This contrasted with the County Court judge who had held that there was no contributory negligence.

Indirect liability of the employer (vicarious liability)

As well as being directly liable for failures to take reasonable care of the health and safety of the employee, an employer is also indirectly liable for negligence of employees who are acting in the course of employment. This concept of vicarious liability means that the employer would have to pay compensation to a person injured as a result of negligence by employees, even though the employer was not itself at fault. Vicarious liability ensures that the innocent victim obtains compensation from the employer, who is required to be compulsorily insured, although the Employer's Liability (Compulsory Insurance) Act does not apply to NHS organisations. A recent House of Lords decision has extended the concept of vicarious liability beyond a narrow meaning of 'course of employment'. The owner and manager of a residential school for maladjusted boys was held vicariously liable for the actions of a warden at the school who had been convicted of serious sexual and physical assaults on the claimants who sought compensation from the defendant. The House of Lords concentrated on the relative closeness of the connection between the nature of the employment and the particular wrong committed by the employee. It was considered fair and just to hold the defendant vicariously liable for the warden's wrongful acts, which had to be deemed to be done in the course of his employment on the basis that those acts were done in an unauthorised and improper mode (*Lister v. Hesley Hall* [2001]).

Application of the law to *Scenario 5.1*

Violet is an employee of Roger Park NHS Trust. She, therefore, has a contract of employment into which the law will imply certain terms. One of these terms is that her Trust owes her a duty to take reasonable care of her health and safety. If Violet can show that the Trust (or one of its employees for which the Trust is vicariously liable) has been at fault in failing to take reasonable care of her safety, and if Violet can show that it was a consequence of this failure that she has become infected with hepatitis, then she should be able to claim compensation.

Evidence such as the failure by the trust to provide reasonable equipment to prevent cross-infection, perhaps an absence of necessary training in sound cross-infection practices, would all be relevant in the attempt to show that the employer is at fault. Violet will also have to show a causal link between the employer's breaches of contract, or another employee's negligence, and the fact that she has contracted hepatitis B.

Contributory negligence

If Violet were to claim compensation from the Trust, the Trust might defend itself by arguing that Violet was herself at fault and that she was partly or even fully responsible for being infected with hepatitis. For example, it may be able to show that it had provided proper training but that Violet failed to follow basic cross-infection procedures and that she was therefore to blame. This defence is known as a defence of contributory negligence and is provided for by Section 1 of the Law Reform (Contributory Negligence) Act 1945 (*Box 5.1*). The defendant is saying to the claimant: you failed to take care of yourself and that has led to, or increased, the harm that you have suffered. If the judge is satisfied that the defendant has succeeded in this defence, he/she is able to reduce the compensation by the extent to which he/she considers the claimant's fault has contributed to the harm.

The fact that an employee has responsibilities for health and safety implementation does not necessarily mean that Violet could not obtain compensation if she injured herself. For example, an employee with responsibility for health and safety was injured when he knelt and tripped on a bolt left by a fellow employee and fell from a platform sustaining soft tissue injuries to his neck and left shoulder, an injury to his head and left elbow. The employers

---

Box 5.1. Section 1 of the Law Reform (Contributory Negligence) Act 1945

Section 1(i) Where any person suffers damage as the result partly of his own fault and partly of any other person or persons a claim in respect of that damage shall not be defeated by reason of the fault of the person suffering the damage, but the damages recoverable in respect thereof shall be reduced to such an extent as the court thinks just and equitable having regard to the claimant's share in responsibility for the damage.

argued that because he was responsible for health and safety procedures, any breach of relevant legislation was his own fault. The court however held that the health and safety documentation had been carefully and impressively prepared by the claimant. However he could not be expected to supervise employees every minute of the day and there was a duty on all employees to take care of their own safety and that of fellow employees. Whilst the claimant was responsible for the implementation of health and safety procedures, he was not responsible for the presence of the bolt. The bolt's presence amounted to a tripping hazard and thus negligence on the part of the employer was established. However the claimant was held to be one third contributorily negligent for failing to see the bolt before he knelt down (*Sullivan v. HWF Ltd* 2001)

Effect of failures by the employee

Scenario 5.2. Supervision of staff

Petunia was the ward manager of a surgical ward and was concerned that a staff nurse, Avril, was not following the correct principles in dressing the wounds of patients. Her failure to follow basic control of infection techniques was risking contamination of the wound and also infecting herself.

Implied terms of the contract binding on the employee

It follows from the implied terms in the contract relating to the duties of the employee, that where the employee is in breach of these terms, then the employer has the right to take action against the employee. In *Scenario 5.2*, as ward manager, Petunia would have responsibilities to take the appropriate action against Avril. Avril is at fault in not obeying reasonable instructions relating to control of infection practices. She is also at fault in not taking reasonable care in carrying out her work. Petunia should follow the disciplinary procedure in taking action against Avril. It may be initially that only an oral warning is necessary. However, if Avril persists in failing to follow good practice then further disciplinary action, such as a written warning, may be justified. Evidence that the employer had taken breaches of health and safety practice seriously and applied the disciplinary procedure to the employee, would be an important defence to the employer, if the employee were to suffer harm and attempt to obtain compensation from the employer.

Duty to non-employees: The laws of negligence

Even though patients, visitors and others have no contract with an employer, a duty is owed by an organisation to others in the laws of negligence. This duty is comparable to the statutory duty under Section 3 of the Health and Safety at Work Act 1974 which places a general duty upon an employer to

> *...conduct their undertaking in such a way as to ensure, so far as is reasonably practicable, that persons not in their employment who may be affected thereby are not thereby exposed to risks to their health and safety.*
>
> *(Chapter 2)*

In the law of negligence a person who has been injured (or if the individual has died, his or her personal representatives) can bring an action for compensation. The claimant must establish on a balance of probabilities that:

- A duty of care was owed by the defendant to him or her.
- There has been a breach of this duty of care by a failure to comply with a reasonable standard.
- As a reasonably foreseeable consequence of this breach of duty the claimant has suffered harm.

Where a claimant can establish these elements compensation will be payable subject to a possible reduction for contributory negligence (see above).

In determining what was reasonable, the courts take into account such factors as:

- The seriousness of the risk.
- The risk of serious harm.
- The cost and practicability of taking precautions to overcome the risk.
- The object to be achieved.

Where the claimant has been injured on premises he or she was visiting there may also be a claim under the Occupiers' Liability Act 1957 *(Chapter 8)*.

Extent of the employer's duty of care to others

The High Court has held that an employer had a duty of care to take reasonable care not to expose the wives of their employees to the risk of injury to their health consequent on their exposure to asbestos dust brought home each working day on the workers' clothes (*Maguire v. Harland and Wolff plc and another* 2004). Mrs Maguire was diagnosed with mesothelioma which resulted from the asbestos dust on her husband's clothes. The employers accepted they were in breach of their duty to the husband, but denied that they owed the wife any duty of care, since it was not foreseeable that she was at risk having regard to her exposure to asbestos dust and the state of knowledge of the risk at the time. The judge held that the risks of serious injury to the wife's health was reasonably foreseeable, and indeed obvious. The defendants had taken no steps to safeguard the wife or her husband from the risk, which could have been reduced by simple and cheap precautions in the context of the cost of shipbuilding and ship-repair contracts. There was no evidence that the defendants ever considered the risk. Reasonably prudent employers should have kept abreast of developing knowledge. A parallel situation in the health care context could be the cross-infection of others by the failure of a health service employer to set up a safe system for decontamination of staff and clothing before leaving hospital premises.

Conclusions

Both employer and employee have contractual duties in relation to health and safety and these are paralleled by the statutory duties under the Health and Safety at Work Act 1974, which were discussed in *Chapter 2*. The statutory duties are enforced through the criminal courts, the contractual duties are enforced through the civil courts (see *Chapter 1* for an explanation of these terms). If an employee has been dismissed following an allegation of a failure to co-operate with the employer in following health and safety requirements or the employee is claiming constructive dismissal, because of a fundamental breach by the employer in fulfilling its contractual duty to take reasonable care of the employee's health and safety, then a hearing may take place in the employment tribunal to consider if there has been an unfair dismissal.

References

Doherty and others v. Rugby Joinery (UK) Ltd 2004 The Times Law Report 3 March 2004

Fraser v. Winchester Health Authority The Times Law Report 12 July 1999

Lister v. Hesley Hall [2001] 2 All ER 769 HL

Maguire v. Harland and Wolff plc and another 2004 The Times Law Report 29 April 2004 QBD

Sullivan v. HWF Ltd (2001) Current Law October 283

Wilsons and Clyde Coal Co Ltd v. English [1937] 3 All ER 628

CHAPTER 6

Remedies for injured employees

Scenario 6.1. Sharp injuries

Angela, a health care assistant who worked in the operating theatre, was severely injured by a scalpel thrown into the bin that was meant for operating theatre linen. This is a common problem faced by the theatre employees who have made frequent complaints about the dangers. What is the law?

Introduction

An employee injured at work will probably wish to claim compensation. Compensation may be claimed under various legal actions, and the burden will usually be placed upon the employee to establish the harm which has been suffered and his/her entitlement. In addition, there are various statutory benefits payable under our social security system for sickness, incapacity and loss of income. Compensation for injuries caused by criminal actions is also payable and this is considered in *Chapter 7*. This chapter considers the remedies that are available to an employee who is injured at work under the Health and Safety Act 1974 and against the employer for breach of contract.

Breach of contract

The employer has an implied duty in the contract of employment that it will take reasonable care of the health and safety of the employee. These contractual duties were considered in *Chapter 5*. The employer's duty covers the duty to take reasonable care to appoint competent staff, and provide safe premises, plant and equipment and a safe system of work. If the employer is in breach of this contractual duty, and as a consequence the employee is injured, then the employee can sue in respect of the harm which he/she has suffered. If the employee is killed as a result of failure by the employer, then the estate of the dead employee can sue for compensation in respect of that death (but the amount payable is fixed by statute and is currently £11 800 for deaths since 1 January 2008), and dependants of the deceased have the right to sue for compensation for the loss of their dependency under the fatal accidents legislation.

As the duty of the employer is to take reasonable care of the health and safety of the employee, there will be situations where an employee is injured but would be unable to recover compensation from the employer because the employer has taken reasonable care. In contrast, if there was an absolute duty placed upon the employer, i.e. strict liability, compensation would be payable whatever the circumstances. Taking reasonable care means that the time, cost and value of any precautions which the employer could take would be relevant to the decision as to what was reasonable for the employer to do.

Negligence

Where an employee has been harmed at work as well as suing for breach of contrast he or she can also sue for breach of the duty of care owed by the employer to the employee in the law of negligence. The employee would have to establish:

- the duty of care,
- the fact that it had been breached, and that
- this breach had caused reasonably foreseeable harm.

In establishing the breach of the duty, the employee would endeavour to show what should have been the standard of care that the employer should have followed. Thus in *Scenario 6.1*, Angela could point to the EU Directive on sharps which came into force in June 2010 giving 3 years for it to be implemented (EU Directive COM 2009 577) and to guidance on the care of sharps issued by the MHRA or by the NPSA or HSE. (Free workshops were organised by Partnership for Occupational Safety and Health in Healthcare on the EU Directive since it was felt that there was limited awareness of the Directive and a number of healthcare organisations were not taking appropriate steps to prevent sharp injuries. The Directive is considered in *Chapter 11*.)

Several employers involved

In 2002, the House of Lords (*Fairchild and others v. Glenhaven Funeral Services Ltd and others* [2002]) held that where several employers were implicated in exposing employees to asbestos dust and fibres, the injured employee did not have to establish which particular employer caused the harm. It was sufficient for the employee to prove that he had been exposed to the inhalation of asbestos dust or fibres and that the employer was in breach of its duty to protect the employee from such risk during different periods of employment. Proof that each employer's wrongdoing had materially increased the risk of contracting the disease was sufficient to satisfy the causal requirements for liability.

This is a significant decision for employees: while they will still have to show that there has been a breach of the duty of care by the employer and that this materially increased the risk of harm to the employee, the employee will not actually have to prove that it was the particular exposure caused by one specific employer which caused the onset of the disease.

Manual handling

In a case in 2002, a nurse, aged 36 years, an employee at Newham General Hospital, who had seriously injured her back by lifting patients, was awarded £420 000 by the High Court (*The Times* 2002). The employer was liable because it had failed to fulfil its responsibilities for her health and safety. The topic of manual handling is considered in *Chapter 9*.

Contributory negligence

Where an employee is partly to blame for the injury, the employer may use the defence known as contributory negligence. In effect, the employer would be arguing that the employee has a duty to care for him/herself and is in breach of this duty and this breach has contributed to the harm that has been suffered (*Chapter 5*). For example, a nurse may be injured when moving a patient. The employers may have been at fault in failing to provide the appropriate equipment for moving patients, but the nurse may have been at fault in not following the instructions on manual handling which he/she was taught in manual handling seminars. In a situation where there is fault on the part of the employer, but also on the part of the employee, and both of these faults lead to the injury suffered, the compensation, to which the employee would be entitled, is reduced to reflect the employee's responsibility for the harm (The Law Reform (Contributory Negligence) Act 1945, *Chapter 5*). An example of the working of the Act can be seen in claims following road traffic accidents. The compensation payable to injured persons, who were not responsible for the accident but were not wearing a seat belt at the time of the accident, may be reduced by about 20 percent. The defence would have to prove that failure to wear a seat belt caused greater injuries to the victim than he or she would have suffered had they been wearing a seat belt.

Willing acceptance of the risk of harm (*volenti non fit injuria*)

In the past it has been argued that in some occupations there is a higher risk of injury and therefore the employee willingly accepts the risk of being injured. However, this defence would not succeed if an employer has failed to take reasonable care of the employee. For example, in *Scenario 6.1*, the fact that being injured by sharps was a known risk in Angela's work would not be a defence to an employer if there was reasonable action which could have been taken to prevent the injury.

Out of time

The claimant must ensure that he or she brings the action within the time limits laid down by the Limitation Acts. Within three years of the injury taking place or the claimant becoming aware of the injury or should have been aware, the claim form must be issued. (The claim form was originally known as the writ.) There are exceptions where the claimant was under a mental disability or where the claimant was under 18 years, in which case the action must be initiated within three years of the disability ending or the child reaching 18 years. The judge also has a discretion to waive the time restriction where it would be just and equitable to do so.

Statutory rights

Under Section 47 of the Health and Safety at Work Act 1974, breach of the main statutory duties (i.e. Sections 2–8) does not give a right to sue for compensation. The reason for this is that the statute creates duties which are enforceable in the criminal courts through prosecutions of employers or employees. However, this may not present a difficulty, since evidence of a criminal conviction can be used in the civil courts and, under Section 11 of the Civil Evidence Act 1968, can be used to show that the guilty person is liable to pay compensation. In addition, breach of the main duties under the 1974 Act may also constitute a breach of contractual duties. In contrast with the general duties under the Act, breach of the regulations may give the right as the basis for a civil action for compensation. For example, a breach of Section 2 of the Health and Safety at Work Act 1974, which places a duty on every employer to ensure, so far as is reasonably practicable, the health, safety and welfare at work of all his/her employees, cannot be used as the basis for a civil action and is enforced through the criminal courts. In contrast, a breach of the Manual Handling Regulations 1992 can be used as evidence of a failure by an employer to take reasonable care of the employee's health and safety.

Dispute over quantum (amount of compensation)

Cases may arise where the employer accepts that it is liable for the harm that an employee has suffered as a consequence of breach of the implied term in the contract of employment for the employer to take reasonable care of the health and safety of the employee. Yet the employer disputes the amount of compensation claimed by the employee. In such a situation, there may be a court hearing on the amount of compensation claimed. It is likely that the employer would have offered the employee a specific amount and if this was refused, paid this sum into court. This amount is kept secret from the judge who would then rule on liability (if this had not been admitted) and on the amount of compensation payable (this amount would be nil, if there were no liability). If the judge's award is less or equal to the sum paid into court by the defendant, then the usual rule is that the claimant pays the costs of both parties which have been incurred from the date of payment-in, since had the payment-in been accepted, there would have been no necessity for a court hearing. It may happen that the costs of the case exceed the amount of the award.

Criminal injury compensation through the criminal courts

In the event of a successful conviction for a criminal offence, the court has the power, in addition to any penalty imposed upon the defendant, to award compensation to a person injured as a result of the criminal offence. The amount awarded will depend upon the court's estimate of the resources of the defendant and the nature of the offence. In the case of *Pola v. The Crown (Health and Safety Executive)* [2009] the injured employee was awarded £90 000 for brain injuries. The case is considered in *Chapter 2*.

Constructive dismissal

Employees who are aware of dangers in the workplace and who do not want to wait until they have been injured to claim compensation may be able to claim constructive dismissal. If dangers are pointed out to an employer who fails to take reasonable action to remedy the situation, then the employer is in fundamental breach of the contract of employment with the employee. This breach of contract by the employer gives the employee the right of election: either to see the contract as at an end and bring an action for unfair dismissal or to see the contract as continuing but seek compensation for breach of contract. The House of Lords has held that where an employee is claiming for unfair dismissal (which includes constructive dismissal) in an employment tribunal, the tribunal cannot award compensation for injury to feelings and pride (and other non-economic loss), but can only award compensation for economic loss according to the statutory provisions of the Employment Rights Act 1996 (*Dunnachie v. Kingston upon Hull City Council* 2004).

Whistle-blowing

The preferred route for an employee to take to secure improvements in the working environment and the removal of dangers is through following the procedure which should have been set up by the employer under the Public Interest Disclosure Act 1998. This is considered in more detail in *Chapter 23*. The legislation provides protection from victimisation for any employee who has brought concerns to the attention of senior management.

Application of the law to the *Scenario 6.1*

Angela and her colleagues have complained about this risk of harm, yet no action has been taken. What action would it be reasonable for the employer to take? More stringent precautions should be taken in the operating theatres to prevent scalpels being mixed with laundry. A count of scalpels used and a check to ensure that they are all accounted for after each operation should be routine procedure. A metal detector for each bag of laundry may prove a simple, reasonable, cheap and effective measure to protect staff from being injured by scalpels. Failure to take such reasonable action may constitute a fundamental breach of contract by Angela's employer. Angela and her colleagues have the right to claim that their employer's failure to take reasonable care of their health and safety gives them the right to see their contract as at an end. They have the right to elect to regard the employer's fundamental breach of contract as in effect ending the contract of employment with them.

This ending of the contract, known as a constructive dismissal, gives employees the right to claim remedies for unfair dismissal. The application would be made to an employment tribunal where the first issue to be determined would be whether the employee has resigned or whether there has been a constructive dismissal. If the latter is established (and clearly the employee would have to provide evidence of the fundamental breach of contract by the employer and the employee's election to regard this as ending the contract), then the tribunal will determine whether the dismissal was unfair, and if so, the compensation payable by the employer and whether an order for reinstatement should be made.

Alternatively or in addition, Angela could seek compensation for the injury to her hand by claiming against the employer for its failure to take reasonable care of her health and safety. Her claim could include compensation for any pain and suffering, any loss in the use of her hand, lost of income and any specific losses she has incurred, e.g. costs in travelling to hospital for her hand to be cared for.

Conclusion

The aim of health and safety laws are to prevent injuries to employees by creating a safe working environment. Safety inspectors and safety committees should be working with employers and employees to identify dangers and ensure reasonable action is taken to protect employees and others (*Chapter 3*). The management of health and safety at work regulations, which were updated and published in 1999 (Statutory Instrument, 1999), place a statutory duty upon the employer to make a risk assessment and take action to remove identified risks as far as is reasonably practicable. Inevitably, however, employees are injured and rely upon the recognised legal actions in the civil courts to obtain compensation. Recommendations have been made by Lord Jackson in his review on civil litigation costs which was published in 2010. These are intended to reduce the growth in civil litigation and make the existing system of no-win, no-fee (whereby an agreement between claimant and solicitor enables a claim to be brought without fear of costs payable by the claimant) less attractive. Legislation is to be introduced. (See also Lord Young's report discussed in *Chapter 24.*) An alternative route may be to seek compensation from the Criminal Injury Compensation Authority (CICA) which will be considered in the next chapter.

References

Dunnachie v. Kingston upon Hull City Council 2004 The Times Law Report 16 July 2004

Fairchild v. Glenhaven Funeral Services Ltd and others; Fox v. Spousal (Midlands) Ltd; Matthews v. Associated Portland Cement Manufacturers Ltd and another (1978) The Times Law Report 21 June 2002; [2002] UKHL 22

Lord Jackson (2010) *Review of Civil Litigation Costs: Final Report.* The Stationery Office, London

Pola v. The Crown (Health and Safety Executive) [2009] EWCA Crim 655

The Times (2002) News item. *The Times*, 17 October

Statutory Instrument (1999) *Management of Health and Safety at Work Regulations. No 3242.* The Stationery Office, London

CHAPTER 7

Criminal injury compensation

Scenario 7.1. Violence in Accident & Emergency

Bob was a staff nurse in the accident and emergency department and was used to dealing with drunk people at weekends. One Friday night, however, he was caring for a patient who had been knocked down by a car. The man's friends were extremely drunk and attempted to interfere with their friend's treatment. Bob asked them to leave, but they refused. He warned them that he would be calling the police but one of them lunged at Bob, who fell backwards against a trolley causing a severe back injury. He was off work for several weeks and was warned that he might never fully recover. How can he obtain compensation?

Introduction

In the last chapter the various ways in which an injured employee can claim compensation were considered. These include suing the employer for breach of its contractual duty to take reasonable care of the health and safety of the employee. Alternatively, if criminal prosecutions take place the employee may be awarded criminal damages by the criminal courts. An alternative route may be to seek compensation from the Criminal Injury Compensation Authority (CICA).

This chapter considers the scheme for obtaining compensation when injury or death follows a violent act and discusses its application to violence within the NHS.

Criminal Injuries Compensation Authority

The CICA is a statutory authority set up under the Criminal Injuries Compensation Act 1995. Details of the current scheme, which has been in operation since November 2008 replacing the scheme which came into effect in April 2001, are available from the CICA headquarters in Glasgow (CICA 2008). Under the 2008 scheme compensation is payable to victims of criminal injuries which are defined as:

- A crime of violence (including arson, fire-raising or an act of poisoning); or
- An offence of trespass on a railway; or
- The apprehension or attempted apprehension of an offender or a suspected offender, the prevention or attempted prevention of an offence, or the giving of help to any constable who is engaged in any such activity.

Most injuries sustained in health and safety incidents such as manual handling, stress and substances hazardous to health would not be seen as the result of crimes of violence.

The CICA determines whether payments are to be made to victims of criminal acts. Those eligible (and these include the victims of crime as well as the dependants of homicide victims) must have reported the crime to the police as soon as possible. The application should be made within two years of the incident, but exceptions can be made to both these requirements.

In the case of *Tait, R (on the application of) v. Criminal Injuries Compensation Appeals Panel* [2009] a policeman won his appeal against the decision of a CICA appeals panel that he was not eligible to receive compensation. His injuries had occurred in a police chase where the criminals deliberately rammed the police car to make their escape. The High Court held that this showed intention to injure the occupants of the car so that it came within the 2001 scheme.

Payments are made against a tariff system up to a maximum of £500000 (paragraph 24 of the scheme), and include:

- Medical expenses.
- Mental health expenses.
- Lost wages for disabled victims (but not for the first 28 full weeks of lost earnings or earning capacity).
- Lost support for dependants of homicide victims.
- Funerals.
- Travel.
- Rehabilitation for disabled victims.
- Pain and suffering.
- Bereavement.
- Loss of parental services.

Procedure for claiming

The procedure is for an application form (available from the CICA, local victim support schemes, Crown court witness service, local police stations or local citizen advice bureaux) to be completed and sent to the CICA. Claim officers at the CICA initially consider the claim to determine whether it comes within the scheme's eligibility criteria. The claim will either be rejected or an offer will be made to the claimant. Once the CICA is notified that the offer has been accepted, the compensation will be paid. In certain circumstances an interim award may be made with the final award awaiting further details, e.g. of the victim's prognosis. Claimants may be asked to attend a centre for medical examination. A claimant has the right to contest the result of the review by appealing to the Criminal Injuries Compensation Appeals Panel. The appellant has 90 days from the date of the notification of the decision within which to appeal to the panel, which is independent of the CICA itself. There is no appeal against the decision of the panel. The CICA can itself reopen a case after its final decision has been made if the medical condition has deteriorated to such an extent that it would be unjust to keep to the original award (paragraphs 56 and 57 of the scheme). The applicant can also seek judicial review of a decision of the CICA (see below).

The tariff

There is a scale of payments covering 25 levels which relate to the kind of injury sustained; level one is the minimum claim payable and is set at £1000, and level 25 is set at £250000. Level 25 includes quadriplegia/tetraplegia. Level 1 covers multiple minor injuries or disabling but temporary mental anxiety lasting more than six weeks and medically verified. Where compensatable injuries come under several different levels, the highest level award is paid out for the highest rated injury, and then 30% of the tariff for the next serious injury, and 15% of the tariff for the next serious injury.

Withholding of compensation

The scheme permits compensation to be refused if claimants have a criminal record or if their conduct led to them being injured. In addition, people who fail to co-operate in bringing an offender to justice may be refused compensation. The CICA has discretion to withhold or reduce an award on these grounds. Paragraph 13 of the 2008 scheme sets out reasons which would justify the withholding or reduction of an award because of the claimant's conduct. Where the assailant and victim were sharing the same household, payment will not be made if the assailant would benefit or if they are still living together. This applies to a man and woman living together whether they are or are not married and a same sex couple whether or not they are in a civil partnership.

Application to situations in health care

The criminal injury compensation scheme is designed to provide compensation following a crime of violence. Thus, for example, a person can only obtain compensation if injured in a road traffic accident if the vehicle was used as a weapon. The CICA has to be satisfied that the driver deliberately drove it at the claimant in an attempt to cause injury. There is no legal definition of the term 'crime of violence', but the guidance suggests that crimes of violence would usually involve a physical attack on the person.

In a psychiatric hospital, if a patient assaulted a member of staff and caused injury, this should be reported to the police and, if the harm suffered comes within the minimum requirement of the scheme, compensation should be payable. Similarly, if health care employees are injured by patients or visitors, a report should be made to the police and an application made to the CICA. Even where the incident would not result in a criminal conviction, compensation may be payable. For example, where a psychiatric patient has harmed another person, a prosecution against the patient may fail on the grounds that the patient was incapable of forming the mental element required in a crime of assault or grievous bodily harm. Similarly, if the injury was caused by aggression from a child who was below the age of criminal culpability and could not be convicted of a criminal offence, the victim might still be eligible for compensation. Paragraph 10 of the 2008 scheme states that:

> ...even where the injury is attributable to conduct within paragraph 8 (e.g. crime of violence) in respect of which the assailant cannot be convicted of an offence by reason of age, insanity or diplomatic immunity, the conduct may nevertheless be treated as constituting a criminal act.

Under the original scheme, train drivers who had suffered traumatic stress disorder as a result of a person committing suicide on the line were refused compensation because a criminal offence had not been committed. The 2001 and 2008 schemes provide compensation for an employee of a railway company who sees a person injured or killed as a result of trespassing on the railway. The shock suffered must be sufficiently serious to qualify under at least the lowest tariff level.

Community health professionals who are faced with dangerous animals may also be eligible for compensation if they are attacked by a dog. However, the CICA would have to be satisfied that the attack amounted to a crime of violence before being prepared to consider making an award. Compensation may be considered if the person in charge of the dog deliberately set the dog on the health professional or the attack was the result of the dog owner's failure to control an animal which was known to be vicious towards humans and the lack of control amounted to recklessness and a criminal act.

Reforms

A report by the Comptroller and Auditor General investigated the functioning of the CICA and reported to the House of Commons (Home Office 2000). It made significant recommendations: to improve the recruitment and selection of staff; to provide more support and information to applicants (particularly on eligibility); to monitor the characteristics of applicants (especially their ethnicity to establish if there are differences in application rates between different ethnic groups); and to improve quality assurance mechanisms. It also suggested improvements in the processing of applications and suggested that a telephone call centre should be set up. As a consequence of these recommendations, the scheme was established in April 2001 and updated in 2008. Information relating to the CICA should be available to all NHS staff, who should ensure that if they are injured at work a check is made on their eligibility to receive compensation.

Judicial review of CICA decisions and actions

The High Court held that the CICA has a duty to hear a claim for compensation within a reasonable time after receiving all the evidence it said it would need in order to determine the claim (*R (H) v. Criminal Injuries Compensation Authority*, 2002). The remedy of the claimant in the above case was initially to ask the court to order the CICA to determine the claim by a certain date, rather than apply for damages under Article 6 of the European Convention of Human Rights. In the case the court ordered the CICA to determine the claim within 28 days.

In another case (*The Times* 2004a) a woman won her High Court case for judicial review of her criminal injuries compensation claim after suffering sex abuse while in foster care. The woman, aged 37, said that she was abused by her foster mother's son in Blackpool between 1979 and 1981 which caused her serious psychological damage. The Criminal Injuries Compensation Authority was to reconsider the case. In another case the CICA won (*The Times* 2004b). It had refused compensation to a 13-year-old girl who had had sex with an older man on the grounds that she had consented. The girl sought judicial review in the High Court, but the judge pointed to the girl's claims of previous sexual experience and rejected her claim that she had been the victim of violence. The man had pleaded guilty to unlawful sexual intercourse and had been sentenced to a year's imprisonment.

Re-opening of CICA award

A claims officer may re-open a case where there has been such a material change in the victim's medical condition that injustice would occur if the original assessment of compensation were allowed to stand, or where the victim has since died in consequence of the injury. Normally this cannot take place more than two years after the final decision on the award. However the claims officer can extend this two-year limit if he is satisfied, on the basis of evidence presented in support of the application to re-open the case, that the renewed application can be considered without a need for further extensive enquiries.

In the case of *Criminal Injuries Compensation Authority v Criminal Injuries Compensation Appeals Panel & Anor* [2010] the CICA appealed against the overruling of a decision by the Adjudicator that an application by a recipient of criminal injury compensation could not have her award reopened. The facts were that Mrs Lamb was attacked and injured in a car park and received £2500 from the CICA as compensation for a strained back. She subsequently requested that the award should be reviewed in the light of subsequent psychological harm that she had suffered. The Adjudicator ruled that she had suffered psychological problems before the violence and therefore the award could not be reviewed. She sought judicial review of this decision and succeeded. The CICA appealed but the Court of Appeal dismissed the appeal holding that:

- Her current psychiatric condition showed that she was suffering from florid symptoms associated with post-traumatic stress disorder.
- This condition was directly attributable to the assault.
- This represented a material change in her psychiatric condition since the hearing in March 1999.

Application of the law to *Scenario 7.1*

Bob has clearly been the victim of a criminal offence. He should ensure that a report is made to the police. The victim should personally ensure that the police are notified of the offence. The CICA considers that it is not sufficient for a report to be made by a friend, relative or workmate and it would not normally accept reports made to employers, trade union officials or social workers as sufficient. However, in the case of injuries sustained in mental hospitals and prisons, it accepts that a prompt report to the appropriate person in authority represents a willingness that the matter should be formally investigated. Bob's manager should encourage a public prosecution of the offender under the 'zero tolerance' policy towards violence in health care (*Chapter 21*) instituted by the Secretary of Health (Department of Health 2001). Bob may also find that if the offender is prosecuted and convicted, the judge may order criminal compensation to be paid by the defendant. Any payment from another source would be taken in account by the CICA in its award. The tariff for back injuries ranges from £1000 (level one) for a strained back that is disabling for six to 13 weeks, to £11000 (level 13) for ruptured intervertebral disc(s) requiring surgical removal or permanent seriously disabling strained back. It will be noted how small these amounts are in comparison with some of the awards made by the civil courts in actions relating to back injuries at work where negligence can be established.

Conclusion

Most employees who have been injured at work, even though the injuries may be the result of a criminal offence under the Health and Safety at Work Act 1974, would not be eligible for compensation under the CICA scheme since these health and safety crimes are not crimes of violence. However, injuries caused by the aggression of patients, visitors and others will probably come within the scheme. It is important that the appropriate report is made to the police as soon as possible and that the injured employee receives all the necessary support and guidance from health and safety officers, human resource departments and managers.

References

Criminal Injuries Compensation Authority (CICA) (2008) *Criminal Injuries Compensation Scheme*. CICA, Glasgow

Criminal Injuries Compensation Authority v. Criminal Injuries Compensation Appeals Panel & Anor [2010] EWCA Civ 1433

Department of Health (2001) *Violence Against NHS Staff 'Will not be Tolerated'*. Press release. Department of Health, London

Home Office (2000) *Compensating Victims of Violent Crime*. Report by the Comptroller and Auditor General. Home Office, London

R (H) v. Criminal Injuries Compensation Authority (2002) The Times 25 November

Tait, R (on the application of) v. Criminal Injuries Compensation Appeals Panel [2009] EWHC 767 (Admin)

The Times (2004a) News item. Sex abuse claim. *The Times*, 13 July

The Times (2004b) Girl who enjoyed sex refused payout. *The Times* 13 July

Criminal Injuries Compensation Authority (CICA) Glasgow (headquarters): CICA Tay House, 300 Bath Street, Glasgow G2 4LN. Freephone: 0800 358 3601; Fax: 0141 331-2287

CHAPTER 8

Occupiers' Liability Act 1957

> ### Scenario 8.1. A home visit
>
> Aubretia was a physiotherapist working for the Roger Park Hospital and her list of patients included some who lived on a very deprived estate. She was visiting one elderly person when she fell through a rotten floorboard and sustained severe injuries to her leg. She was admitted to hospital and was off work for several weeks. She is anxious to obtain compensation and seeks legal advice.

Introduction

This chapter considers the provisions of the Occupiers' Liability Act 1957, its application to health care and non-health care premises, the duties of the occupier and the rights of the visitor.

Occupiers' Liability Act 1957

An occupier (or owner) of premises has a statutory duty to ensure that visitors to his/her premises are safe. Therefore, where a visitor suffers an injury resulting from the state of the premises the visitor may be able to bring a legal action for compensation against the occupier or owner. The person must be visiting the premises with the express or implied consent of the occupier. The statutory duty to ensure that the premises are safe is placed upon the occupier by the Occupiers' Liability Act 1957. The statutory duty is set out in *Box 8.1*. In *Box 8.1* it will be noted that the duty owed by the occupier to the visitor is a 'reasonable' duty. This means that if the occupier can show that he/she took all reasonable steps to safeguard the safety of the visitor, then the visitor may not be able to recover compensation for any harm suffered

The occupier's duty to trespassers comes under the Occupiers' Liability Act 1984 which is considered in the next chapter.

Box 8.1. Statutory duty of the occupier under Occupiers' Liability Act 1957

- Section 2(1): An occupier of premises owes the same duty, the 'common duty of care', to all his visitors, except in so far as he is free to and does extend, restrict, modify or exclude his duty to any visitor or visitors by agreement or otherwise
- Section 2(2): The common duty of care is a duty to take such care, as in all the circumstances of the case is reasonable, to see that the visitor will be reasonably safe in using the premises for the purposes for which he is invited or permitted by the occupier to be there

---

Visitor

The duty under the Occupiers' Liability Act 1957 is owed to the visitor. This term 'visitor' includes the person who has expressed permission to be on the premises as well as the person who has implied permission to be on the premises. In the hospital context, the term 'visitors' will include employees, patients, friends and relatives visiting patients, contractors and suppliers, and others who have a genuine interest in being in the hospital. If any of these persons were to be injured, e.g. if plaster fell off the wall, they could claim compensation from the occupier.

Not all of these persons will have had an express invitation to be on the premises. As long as they are there with the implicit agreement of the occupier, they would be considered to be visitors. However, at any time the occupier can withdraw this implied consent to be on the premises, and that person would then become a trespasser, if he/she fails to leave.

The occupier

The occupier is the person who has control over the premises. This will usually be the owner of the premises, but not necessarily. There could be several occupiers, each having control over the premises and responsibilities for the safety of the building. For example, contractors might be working on hospital premises and both the NHS trust and the contractor could be regarded as occupiers for the purpose of the Act. A private house visited by a community nurse may be owner-occupied, in which case that person will be the occupier for the purposes of the Act. Alternatively, it could be under a tenancy agreement, in which case the landlord and the tenant will have different duties under this agreement regarding the upkeep and maintenance of the premises and both could therefore be regarded as occupiers under the statutory provisions. Which occupier is liable for harm to a visitor will therefore depend upon the cause of the injury.

Examples of decided cases

A visitor slipped on polish that had been put on the floor but not wiped off, which left the floor excessively slippery. The visitor succeeded in obtaining compensation for the harm. The occupier had failed to take reasonable care for the safety of the visitor (this was a case decided before the 1957 Act, but the result would be the same after 1957) (*Slade v. Battersea HMC* [1955]). It will be expected that the visitor will take reasonable care for him/herself as is shown in a more recent case (*Dobell v. Thanet DC* 1999), where the injured person failed to obtain compensation. A woman sustained personal injuries when, late at night, she fell down a flight of stairs leading to a public lavatory for which the local authority (in this case Thanet District Council) was responsible. The premises were locked and the stairway was unlit. She admitted that she had drunk a relatively small amount of alcohol. She sued the local authority on the grounds that they were occupiers of the premises and owed a duty of care to her. She lost the case on the grounds that she had voluntarily accepted the risk of injury by using the stairs in the darkness and without taking proper care for her own safety. Further, the evidence from the accident and emergency department showed that she had consumed a greater amount of alcohol than she had admitted in evidence. Even if the court was wrong on the voluntary assumption of risk, she would be contributorily negligent to a high degree.

In another case, a woman who slipped on a mushroom in a supermarket and was left wheelchair bound following the accident, was awarded £500000. Asda had accepted liability but disputed the amount of compensation (Fresco 2003).

Warning notice

Section 2(4)(a) of the Occupiers' Liability Act 1957 is set out in *Box 8.2*. The warning is not conclusive: if compliance with it is sufficient to prevent any harm to the visitor, then it will be effective as a defence in an action under the 1957 Act.

Box 8.2. Warning notice

- Section 2(4) In determining whether the occupier of premises has discharged the common duty of care to a visitor, regard is to be had to all these circumstances, so that (for example)
- 2(4)(a): where damage is caused to a visitor by a danger of which he had been warned by the occupier, the warning is not to be treated without more as absolving the occupier from liability, unless in all the circumstances it was enough to enable the visitor to be reasonably safe

---

Scenario 8.2. An adequate notice?

The surgical wards of an NHS trust are being upgraded and a notice is placed at the entrance which says 'Danger – major upgrade'. Occupational therapist Jane Black enters the ward and trips over a ladder which is leaning against a wall. She suffers a severe injury to her ankle and is off sick for several weeks.

In the situation in *Scenario 8.2*, if there were other precautions that the NHS trust could reasonably have taken, e.g. a safety net cordoning off the work area, then the NHS trust would probably be seen to have been in breach of its duty of care to the occupational therapist, subject to the possibility of contributory negligence by her. If, on the other hand, the notice said 'entrance closed, follow diversion' and indicated a different route which was practicable, then the occupier would have satisfied the duty under the Act.

If the occupational therapist ignored the notice, failed to look out for the ladder and was injured, then it is probable that there would be no breach of duty by the NHS trust since the notice was in all the circumstances enough to enable the occupational therapist to be reasonably safe. If the ladder was left there by independent contractors (see below), then that firm could be seen as occupiers for the purposes of the Act and may be liable, subject to the care or lack of care taken by the occupational therapist.

Independent contractors

Where independent contractors are brought on to site the usual occupier or owner of the premises will not normally be liable for their safety (*Box 8.3*). However the Court of Appeal has held that an occupier of land who engaged an independent contractor to perform a pyrotechnic display on his land owed a duty to ensure that the contractor had adequate public liability insurance cover (*Bottomley v. Secretary and Members of Todmoron Cricket Club and others*). Health service organisations which invite independent contractors on to their premises should ensure that they are adequately insured.

Box 8.3. Liability of an independent contractor

- Section 2(4)(b): When damage is caused to a visitor due to the faulty execution of any work or construction, maintenance or repair by an independent contractor employed by the occupier, the occupier is not to be treated without more as answerable for the danger, if in all the circumstances he had acted reasonably in entrusting the work to an independent contractor and had taken such steps (if any) as he reasonably ought in order to satisfy himself that the contractor was competent and that the work had been properly done

---

Contracted out services

Where services such as cleaning and catering are contracted out, the law relating to independent contractors (*Box 8.3*) will apply. If those firms fail to ensure that the premises are reasonably safe, they could be liable under the Occupiers' Liability Act 1957.

Defective Premises Act 1972

Under this Act where a lease imposes an obligation on the landlord in respect of maintenance and repair of the property then the landlord will be held to owe a duty of care to all those who might reasonably be expected to be affected by any defects in the state of the premises. However, the landlord must know or ought reasonably to have known of the relevant defect and the defect should be one which the landlord should have remedied by virtue of his obligation to repair imposed by the lease. The landlord's duty is owed not only to the tenant but also to any visitors to the premises. The Court of Appeal held that the duty owed by a building contractor under S1 of the Defective Premises Act 1972 to see that work was done in such a manner that the dwelling would be fit for habitation when completed applied only to new building. (*Jenson and Another v. Faux* 2011)

Overlap of statutory provisions

The duty of the occupier under the Occupiers' Liability Act 1957 may overlap with the duties of the employer under Health and Safety at Work legislation and an injured employee could rely on all the different statutory provisions in bringing a case for compensation. Thus, in the case of *Donaldson v. Brighton DC* 2002, a caretaker who used an unsafe ladder to reach a loft succeeded in obtaining compensation for the personal injuries he suffered when he fell off the ladder. The court held that there was a breach of the duty of care owed under the Occupiers' Liability Act 1957; a breach of the Provision and Use of Work Equipment Regulations 1992 (SI 1992 2932) and a breach of the Manual Handling Regulations 1992 (SI 1992 2793). The Occupiers' Liability Act 1957 also overlaps with the common law of negligence under which a duty is owed to individuals who would be harmed by reasonably foreseeable risks. To establish liability under the Occupiers' Liability Acts it will be necessary to establish that there has been a breach of the duty owed and that this breach caused the harm which was suffered, and whether there has been a breach and/or causation are decided by the usual rules of negligence. (See *Chapters 5 and 6* for further details of the law of negligence.)

Application of the law to *Scenario 8.1*

Where health professionals are visiting private homes, the occupier may be the owner of the house who is also in occupation, or the occupier may be a tenant. In *Scenario 8.1* it is likely that the occupier is a tenant, not the owner. Aubretia's injuries relate to the structure of the premises for which the landlord and owner would be liable. In contrast, if she had been injured as the result of a frayed rug or furnishings, for which the tenant was responsible, her claim would have to be made against the tenant. The difficulty is that the tenant is unlikely to be able to pay any compensation or to have the necessary insurance cover. The landlord or owner is more likely to have the necessary cover. Aubretia will be able to obtain statutory benefits for being off sick and incapacitated. She would not be able to seek compensation under the Occupiers' Liability Act 1957 against her employer, since the NHS trust is not the occupier of the premises. Also, it could not be established that Aubretia's injury has been caused as a result of failures by the employer to take reasonable care of the health and safety of its employee (this would only arise if the employers knew that the premises were unsafe to the point of being dangerous and in spite of that knowledge, compelled Aubretia to visit).

If Aubretia had private accident insurance cover, or if her professional association had such cover for its members, then she would be entitled to compensation for personal injury.

Conclusion

Those visitors (including employees) who are injured on NHS premises can claim compensation for injuries arising from the premises and only have to prove that their injuries were caused by the occupier's failure to take reasonable care of the safety of the visitor. Those health professionals who work in the community are vulnerable to the ability of an occupier or owner to meet the cost of liability for harm arising from the premises. The liability of the occupier for children who are visitors will be considered in the next chapter, together with the occupier's liability for trespassers.

References

Bottomley v. Secretary and Members of Todmoron Cricket Club and others Times Law
Report 13 November 2003

Dobell v. Thanet DC (1999) March 22 Current Law August 2000 No 527

Donaldson v. Brighton DC (2002) Current Law Digest 344

Fresco A (2003) £1/2 million for woman who slipped on a mushroom. *The Times,* 24
January

Jenson and Another v. Faux The Times Law Report 26 April 2011

Slade v. Battersea HMC [1955] WLR 207

CHAPTER 9

Occupiers' liability for children and trespassers

Scenario 9.1. Child visitors and trespassers

Violet was a practice nurse and was on duty in a GP health centre when a child who was accompanying his mother wandered unnoticed into the cleaner's room, opened a cupboard door and started drinking from a bottle of bleach. The child suffered considerable harm and the parents wish to obtain compensation from the health centre. What is the legal situation?

Introduction

This chapter considers the liability of the occupier for children who are visitors, together with the occupier's liability for trespassers.

Liability for children under the Occupiers' Liability Act 1957

In the *Chapter 8* we considered the duty owed by the occupier of premises under the Occupiers' Liability Act 1957 to take:

Such care as in all the circumstances of the case is reasonable to see that the visitor will be reasonably safe in using the premises for the purposes for which he is invited or permitted by the occupier to be there.

The 1957 Act expressly provides that all the circumstances must be taken into account in deciding whether the occupier is in breach of his/her duty of care under the Act (*Box 9.1*). The occupier can expect a lower standard of care from children and therefore additional precautions have to be taken where the presence of children can be foreseen.

Box 9.1. Occupiers' Liability Act 1957 Section 2(3)

The circumstances relevant for the present purpose include the degree of care, and of want of care, which would ordinarily be looked for in such a visitor, so that (for example) in proper cases an occupier must be prepared for children to be less careful than adults.

Child injured by falling boat

An example of a situation where children were injured and brought a claim under the Occupiers' Liability Act 1957 is shown in the case set out in *Box 9.2*. The High Court judge awarded the claimant £633770 taking into account contributory negligence of 25% for the injuries sustained by the boy. However, the Court of Appeal found in favour of the defendant since, although it was reasonably foreseeable that injuries could have occurred from playing on the boat, the injuries sustained were not reasonably foreseeable and therefore the defendants were not liable for them. The Council involved in this case had not disputed that it was negligent, but argued that it was not liable because the accident was of a different kind from anything which it could have reasonably foreseen. The claimant appealed to the House of Lords, which upheld the appeal. The House of Lords held that the ingenuity of children in finding unexpected ways of doing mischief to themselves and others should not

---

Box 9.2. *Jolley v. Sutton London Borough Council*

Sutton Borough Council were the owners and occupiers of the common parts of a block of council flats. A boat with trailer was brought onto the land and abandoned on a grass area where children played. The boat became derelict and rotten. The Council put a notice on the boat which said 'Do not touch this vehicle unless you are the owner'. Some boys planned to repair it in the hope that they could take it to Cornwall. They swivelled it round and jacked the front up and put it on to the trailer so as to be able to get under the boat to repair the hull. The boat fell onto the claimant, a boy of 14 years, as he lay underneath it attempting to repair and paint it. He sustained serious spinal injuries and became paraplegic.

---

be underestimated. Reasonable foreseeability was not a fixed point on the scale of probability. The Council was liable under the Occupiers' Liability Act 1957, and under section 2(3) had to take into account the fact that children would be less careful than adults. The Council had admitted that it should have removed the boat, and the risk which it should have taken into account was that children would meddle with the boat and injuries would thereby occur.

Implications for health care

Children may come on to health premises as patients or to accompany patients. They would be regarded as visitors for the purposes of the Occupiers' Liability Act 1957 unless there was express prohibition on bringing children on to the premises. Where children come on to premises as visitors, the occupier has a more stringent duty in relation to their safety and has to expect that children will be less careful than adults. Special precautions must be taken for the safety of children on children's wards, in outpatients clinics, and in accident and emergency and other departments where the presence of children can be anticipated.

Trespassers and the Occupiers' Liability Act 1984

The Occupiers' Liability Act 1957 is not concerned with the liability of the occupier for trespassers. After the 1957 Act was passed, there were several cases involving child trespassers and the courts recognised that a limited duty of the occupier towards trespassers, particularly children, was owed under principles established at common law. The leading case was that of the *British Railway Board v. Herrington* [1972] in which the House of Lords stated that a duty of common humanity was owed by an occupier if he was aware that there were dangers on his land which could be attractive to children who could be harmed thereby.

Subsequently, statutory provision for the occupiers' duty towards trespassers was made in the Occupiers' Liability Act 1984. Whether or not a duty is owed by the occupier to trespassers, in relation to risks on the premises, depends upon the factors set out in section 1(3) (*Box 9.3*).

Duty to trespassers

In applying the factors shown in *Box 9.3* to decide if a duty is owed to a trespasser, it would be rare for a duty to be owed to an adult. However, there is more likely to be recognition that a duty of care is owed to a child trespasser. Thus, for example,

---

Box 9.3. Occupiers' Liability Act 1984 section 1(3)

a. If the occupier is aware of the danger or has reasonable grounds to believe that it exists
b. If the occupier knows or has reasonable grounds to believe that the other is in the vicinity of the danger concerned or that he may come into the vicinity of the danger (in either case, whether the other has lawful authority for being in that vicinity or not)
c. The risk is one against which, in all the circumstances of the case, he may reasonably be expected to offer the other some protection

---

on hospital premises, if a child is expressly told that he/she cannot go through a particular door or into another section of the hospital and the child disobeys those instructions, then he/she becomes a trespasser for the purposes of the Occupiers' Liability Act. A duty may then arise under the 1984 Act.

The nature of the duty owed to trespassers

Once it is held that a duty of care is owed to a trespasser, section 1(4) of the 1984 Act defines the duty as shown in *Box 9.4*. The duty to trespassers under section 1(4) can be discharged by giving warnings (section 1(5)), but in the case of children this may have limited effect and it would depend upon the age of the child. An example of a case where it was held that a duty was owed to a trespasser was the case of *Tomlinson v. Congleton Borough Council and another* (2002) CA. The claimant suffered from appalling injuries when he dived into shallow water in the lake at Brereton Heath Park, Congleton and hit his head on the bottom. The Court of Appeal (by a majority verdict) held that whilst there were prominent signs forbidding swimming and park rangers were employed, they were not sufficient to discharge the council from its duty to take reasonable care to prevent injury to those

---

Box 9.4. Occupiers' Liability Act 1984 section 1(4)

Section 1(4): The duty is to take such care as is reasonable in all the circumstances of the case to see that he (the trespasser) does not suffer injury on the premises by reason of the danger concerned.

---

going into the water. The Council had started planting over the sandy beach to deter swimmers but had not completed this work. The claimant accepted that on entering the water he ceased to be a visitor and became a trespasser. The Court of Appeal held that the Council was in breach of its duty to take reasonable care to see that he did not suffer injury at the park by reason of the dangers which awaited those who entered the water to swim. The claimant was held to be two-thirds contributorily negligent. The dissenting judge Lord Justice Longmore held that there were obvious dangers in going for a swim in any stretch of water other than a dedicated swimming pool. This lake was no different from any other stretch of open water. That the Council promoted the site for leisure activities did not mean that it had to take steps to prevent swimming unless it knew of any particular hazard. Even then to give a warning in relation to such a hazard should probably be sufficient.

The defendants appealed to the House of Lords which allowed the appeal, supporting the dissenting judgment of Lord Longmore in the Court of Appeal. (*Tomlinson v. Congleton* 2002 HL).

It held that the swimmer had no claim under Section 1 of the Occupier's Liability Act 1984. It held that he was a person who had full capacity and had voluntarily engaged in an activity that had the inherent risk that he might not execute his dive properly and so sustain injury. The only risk had arisen out of what he had chosen to do, not out of the state of the premises. There had therefore arisen no risk of the kind that gave rise to a duty under the 1984 Act. The House of Lords held that local authorities and other occupiers of land were ordinarily under no duty to incur such social and financial costs to protect a minority or even a majority against obvious dangers. Interestingly the House of Lords, whilst agreeing that the defendants were not liable, were not agreed on which Act applied. Lord Scott stated that the swimmer had not suffered his injury while swimming. He had run into the water and then executed the disastrous dive. He had, accordingly, not been a trespasser and the relevant act was the 1957 Act rather than the 1984 Act. There had been no breach of duty under the 1957 Act.

Case of *Rhind v. Astbury Water Park Ltd* [2004]

The claimant suffered serious injuries when he dived into a mere to collect his football and hit his head on a concealed fibreglass container. The Court of Appeal rejected his claim under the Occupiers' Liability Act 1984 on the grounds that there were clear notices saying 'Private Property – Strictly no swimming allowed' and he was owed no duty of care under the 1984 Act. The defendants had no knowledge of the container below the surface nor were there reasonable grounds for them to have known.

Refusing to leave premises

The occupier has the right to ask any visitor to leave the premises. Should the visitor fail to leave, then he/she becomes a trespasser and the occupier can use reasonable force to evict the trespasser. Thus, if visitors or patients become aggressive they could be asked to leave by hospital staff. If they refuse to leave, they become trespassers and reasonable force could be used to evict them. Similarly, if a health professional visiting a client in the community was to be asked by a client or carer to leave, he/she should go. Failure to accept the instruction would mean that the health professional would become a trespasser. If the health professional was concerned for the wellbeing of the client, he/she should ensure that social services are notified so that appropriate action can be taken under the National Assistance Act 1948 or the Mental Health Act 1983. Where there is a clash between carer and client and the former asks the health professional to leave and the latter for the health professional to stay, the health professional has to decide on the basis of the specific circumstances – the rights of the client to occupation as compared with those of the carer and the specific needs of the client. Where the health professional considers it prudent to leave the premises, he/she must discuss with his/her manager how best the client's needs can be met.

Application of the law to *Scenario 9.1*

The first question to answer is whether the child in the situation in *Scenario 9.1* is a visitor or a trespasser. If he is held to be the former, then the Occupiers' Liability Act 1957 will apply to him and if he is held to be a trespasser, then the Occupiers' Liability Act 1984 will apply. He certainly came into the health centre as a visitor since even though his mother is the patient, there was an implied permission for her child to accompany her. However, when he moves away from the general areas to which the public is permitted entry and goes into the cleaner's room, he becomes a trespasser. He is certainly not invited or allowed to be on the premises to enter the cleaner's room and is therefore trespassing. The occupier would be the general practitioners who run the practice and/or the primary care trust if it owns the premises.

The next question to be considered is whether the occupier has a duty of care to the child. This can be answered by looking at the situation in the health centre. Should the occupier be aware of the dangers that exist? Are there reasonable grounds for the occupier to believe that the child is or may come into the vicinity of the danger and is the risk one against which, in all the circumstances of the case, the occupier may reasonably offer the trespasser some protection? It would seem that the answer to all these questions is that the occupier should have been aware of the danger and the possibility that an unattended child could access the bleach in the cleaner's room. It could therefore be concluded that the occupier does have a duty of care.

The final question refers to the nature of the duty upon the occupier to this particular trespasser. *Box 9.4* shows that the occupier's duty is to take such care as is reasonable in all the circumstances of the case to see that the child does not suffer injury on the premises by reason of the danger concerned. What reasonable action could the occupiers have taken? Certainly, under the Control of Substances Hazardous to Health (COSHH) regulations (*Chapter 10*) there should have been a risk assessment carried out to identify the risk. To what extent could the GPs have relied upon the parents to exercise supervision of children they bring on to the premises? The parents would have responsibilities to the children, but this might not relieve the GPs of the duty of ensuring that the premises are safe and that any dangerous substances are locked away out of the reach of any wandering children.

Conclusion

There are considerable differences between the occupier's duty to visitors and the duty to trespassers. Reasonable care must be taken over the safety of a visitor. There may, depending upon the circumstances, be no duty owed to a trespasser. However, the younger the child the more likely a duty will exist, but this may well be less onerous than one owed to a visitor. Health organisations and their staff need to ensure that their risk assessments take into account the possible presence of children both as bona fide visitors and as trespassers.

References

British Railway Board v. Herrington [1972] AC 877, 1 All ER 749

Jolley v. Sutton London Borough Council [2000] The Times Law Report 24 May 2000 72 All ER 409

Rhind v Astbury Water Park Ltd [2004] EWCA Civ 756

Tomlinson v. Congleton Borough Council and another (2002) CA Times Law Report 22 March 2002

Tomlinson v. Congleton Borough Council and another (2002) HL Times Law Report 1 August 2003 [2003] UKHL 47

CHAPTER 10

Controlling substances hazardous to health

Scenario 10.1. Dangerous substance

Daisy, the ward manager in the children's ward at Roger Park Hospital, was on duty one morning when she heard a scream and rushed to the cleaner's room. She saw one of the patients with a bottle in his hand clearly in considerable pain and distress. It was subsequently discovered that the boy, aged five years, had wandered from the main ward and found a bottle of cleaning fluid in a cupboard in the cleaner's store room and had taken a drink from it. At the time of the incident, the ward staff had thought that his parents were supervising him.

Introduction

All health workers have responsibilities under the regulations relating to the Control of Substances Hazardous to Health (COSHH). The regulations were first introduced in 1988 but have subsequently been updated (current regulations date from 2002 (SI 2002/2677; amended SI 2004/3386) to implement the more detailed requirements of the EC Chemical Directive (HSE 2002). The health professional who uses different substances in his/her work should be specifically alert to the need to ensure that the regulations are implemented. Where the regulations have not been followed, there can be a prosecution in the criminal courts against the offender. In addition, any person who has been injured as a result of a failure to ensure that reasonable care was taken by the employer would have a right of civil action to claim compensation.

Assessment under COSHH

The HSE (2002 with regular updates) has issued guidance on the implementation of the regulations providing both a 'COSHH in a hurry publication' as well as more detailed guidance on preventing or controlling exposure to hazardous substances at work. The HSE guidance covers: the current legal base; legal developments; key message; the hazardous substances covered by COSHH;

the COSHH requirements; assessing risk; preventing or controlling exposure; ensuring that control measures are used and maintained; monitoring exposure; health surveillance; planning for accidents, incidents and emergencies; and ensuring that employees are properly informed, trained and supervised. It initially recommended an eight-stage assessment. Subsequently the HSE now recommends a five-stage assessment which can be used in relation to any risk to health and safety. These five stages are shown in *Box 10.1*. As part of COSHH assessment the HSE recommends:

1. Walk around your workplace. Where is there potential for exposure to substances that might be hazardous to health?
2. In what way are the substances hazardous to health?
3. What jobs or tasks lead to exposure?
4. Are there any areas of concern, e.g. from the Accident Book?

There must be clarity over who has responsibility for carrying out the assessment, but the guidance emphasises the importance of involving all employees in the assessment.

Box 10.1. Guidance in carrying out a five-step COSHH assessment

1. Identify the hazards
2. Decide who might be harmed and how
3. Evaluate the risk and decide on precaution
4. Record your findings and implement them
5. Review your assessment and update if necessary

Source: HSE, COSHH

Identification of substances and their dangers

The HSE gives guidance on the definition of substances hazardous to health as follows (Health Services Executive 2002 and updated):

COSHH covers chemicals, products containing chemicals, fumes, dusts, vapours, mists and gases, and biological agents (germs). If the packaging has any of the hazard symbols then it is classed as a hazardous substance. COSHH also covers asphyxiating gases; germs that cause diseases such as leptospirosis or legionnaires' disease; and germs used in laboratories.COSHH does not cover lead, asbestos or radioactive substances because these have their own specific regulations.

All potentially hazardous substances must be identified: these will include domestic materials such as bleach, toilet cleaner, window cleaner, and polishes; office materials such as correction fluids; as well as the medicinal products in the treatment room and materials and substances used in the ward or department. An assessment has to be made as to whether each substance could be inhaled, swallowed, absorbed or introduced through the skin, or injected into the body (such as needles). The effects of each route of entry or contact, the potential harm, the persons who could be exposed and how this could occur must then be identified.

Once this assessment is complete, decisions must be made on the necessary measures to be taken to comply with the regulations and who should undertake the different tasks. In certain cases, health surveillance (see below) is required if there is a reasonable likelihood that the disease or ill-effect associated with exposure will occur in the workplace concerned. Health professionals should be vigilant about any substances used in their activities and ensure that a risk assessment is undertaken and its results implemented.

Managers should ensure that employees are given information, instruction and training. Records should show what the results of the assessment are, what action has been taken and by whom, and regular monitoring and review of the situation.

Monitoring

The HSE has provided guidance on monitoring the control of exposure to hazardous substances. The HSE states that monitoring means measuring to show that control is adequate. It has nothing to do with the state of a worker's health. It suggests that monitoring is appropriate:

- when you need to show compliance with a WEL (Workplace Exposure Limit) (see below) or BMGV (Biological Monitoring Guidance Value), and
- when you need to show that control equipment or personal protective equipment is working well enough.

Monitoring can also indicate the spread of contamination, e.g. using surface wipes. Screening, e.g. via colorimetric detector tubes or meters, provides indicators of worker exposure only. Personal air monitoring measures how much of a substance the worker inhales. Biological monitoring measures how much of a substance has entered the body.

Workplace exposure limits

Many thousands of substances are used at work but only about 500 have Workplace Exposure Limits (WELs) listed in *'EH40 Workplace Exposure Limits'*.

The HSE asks, 'How do I know if exposures are below the WEL?' and answers:

You can only do this by monitoring. This means measuring the substance in the air that the worker breathes while the task is under way. A guidance sheet, 'Exposure measurement: Air sampling G409' tells you what to expect from a competent consultant who provides monitoring services.

'What if a hazardous substance has no exposure limit, or it is mixed in a product?'

You can check whether you are using the right control measures. If you are, exposures are likely to be below the WEL. See COSHH EH40 Workplace Exposure Limits table. 'Exposure measurement: Air sampling G409 Working with substances hazardous to health: What you need to know about COSHH'.

Substance substitution

The HSE has provided guidance on substance substitution as follows.
You can prevent exposure to a hazardous substance by:

- Substituting it with another substance which presents less, or no risk; or by
- Using another process which does not create a hazardous form of that substance. For example, substituting a powder for a liquid; removing the need to weigh out powders by buying them pre-packed.

There are seven steps to practical, well-thought-out decisions about substitution.

1. Is the substance or process a hazard?
2. Is there a significant risk involved in storing, using or disposing of a substance?
3. Are there alternatives?
4. What could happen if you use the alternatives? Compare the alternatives with each other and with the substance or process you are using at the moment.
5. Decide whether to substitute.
6. Introduce the substitute.
7. Assess how it is working.

You can speak to trade associations, others carrying out similar work, customers and suppliers for information if you are considering substitution. You should also look at HSE publications.

Training

The HSE gives guidance on training for employees working with substances hazardous to health. This includes providing information and instruction for employees who work with such substances. Cleaning and maintenance staff should be included. The HSE emphasises that employees need to understand the outcome of the employer's risk assessment and what this means for them.

Employers should tell employees:

- What the hazards and risks are;
- About any workplace exposure limit;
- The results of any monitoring of exposure;
- The general results of health surveillance; and
- What to do if there is an accident (e.g. spillage) or emergency.

Employers should keep basic training records.

Employees should have access to safety data sheets. They should be kept informed about planned future changes in the processes or substances used. When contractors come on site, they need to know what the risks are and how the employer is controlling them. The employer needs to know if they are bringing hazardous substances onto the premises, and how they will prevent harm to the employees.

Allergies and COSHH

On 3 May 2000, the Health and Safety Commission held a conference to prepare a draft strategy on occupational asthma. It then published a consultative document in 2000 and a Commission paper in October 2001. It recommended that a target should be set to reduce asthma caused by substances at work and that asthma should be reduced by 30% by 2010. An Asthma Project Board was set up to develop, publish and help implement an action plan on asthma. The revised COSHH regulations 2002 are designed to ensure that any such exposure to employees is prevented.

The Health and Safety Executive has published guidance on general ventilation in the workplace as a means of controlling exposure to substances hazardous to health (HSE 2000).

Failure to provide adequate ventilation: A successful case

An example of a successful case brought in relation to occupational asthma is that of *Ogden v. Airedale Health Authority* [1996]. A radiographer brought the claim against his health authority on the grounds that he was sensitised to X-ray chemicals resulting in occupational asthma and other reversible airways obstruction. He alleged that the sensitisation occurred in the course of his employment as a radiographer at Airedale Hospital and was caused by his employer's negligence and/or breach of statutory duty. The matters relied upon to support his allegations were, failing to:

- Ensure that the environment in which he worked was so far as reasonably practicable free from fumes likely to be harmful to him.
- Regularly monitor his workplaces for such fumes.
- Adequately ventilate the workplaces.
- Provide him with protective equipment (in particular, goggles, masks and an aspirator).
- Warn him of the risk of exposure to fumes.
- Heed or act upon complaints made in 1987 concerning problems of temperature and chemical fumes in the accident and emergency X-ray department of the hospital.

It was also alleged that there were breaches of the COSHH regulations of 1988.

The defendants denied all allegations, including causation and the alleged injuries suffered. They also raised a defence that the claim was out of time, but this was decided in favour of the claimant. The result was that the claimant's case succeeded on the following grounds:

- During the time of the claimant's employment at Airedale Hospital there were in use in his place of work chemicals which were capable of having an irritant effect upon the health of the employees. Some of these chemicals were sensitisers capable of producing skin allergy and asthma and during some of the activities which staff were required to carry out such as the mixing of chemicals there was a likelihood of the recommended exposure limits being exceeded.
- By the time a report was compiled in 1990 the defendants were well aware of the chemical constituents of most but not all of the chemicals in use in the X-ray department of the hospital and of the fact that such chemicals contained irritants and there was a risk of sensitisation.
- The defendants were well aware that their radiographers were complaining that the chemicals used in the department were causing them health problems; during the whole of the claimant's employment at the hospital the defendants knew that the chemicals in use contained irritants.
- If the defendants did not in fact know that the chemicals contained irritants they ought to have done.
- The defendants ought to have taken steps to keep the level of chemical fumes in the X-ray department as low as possible. Their primary strategy should have been to seek to control the fumes at source.
- Until 1988 the defendants did little to safeguard radiography staff at the hospital against the irritant effects of chemicals with which they were working.
- In failing to take the precautions as regards local exhaust ventilation, the provision of protective equipment, the laying down and enforcement of a proper warning system for dealing with spillages, the issuing of warnings to staff as to the hazards associated with X-ray chemicals and the precautions to be taken when handling them, the defendants were guilty of negligence.
- Failure to take such precautions, as they either knew or ought to have known, put the health of the radiographers at risk, and the risk went beyond mere irritation, including the risk of employees becoming sensitised which, if it occurred, might well lead to a radiographer being obliged to give up his/her employment and career as in fact had happened to the claimant.

- The claimant was suffering from occupational asthma induced by exposure to X-ray chemicals and that such exposure was caused by the negligence and breach of statutory duty of the employers.

This case would be relevant to those health practitioners who work in X-ray departments and other areas of the hospital where there are toxic fumes and ventilation problems.

Exposure to latex

In a case brought against an NHS trust (*Dugmore v. Swansea NHS Trust* [2002]), a nurse won her appeal against the dismissal of her claim against her employers. The Court of Appeal held that the trust could not be said to have adequately controlled her exposure to latex given that the nurse was often obliged to wear latex gloves when other types of barrier could have been supplied. The trust had either failed to have knowledge of the risk of allergic reaction to latex gloves or had underestimated the risk and taken no precautions against it. Accordingly, the trust had breached Reg. 7(1) of the 1988 and 1994 COSHH Regulations. Damages were eventually assessed as £350000 including interest of £114193 (de Bruxelles 2004).

In March 2002, the Department of Health announced that new guidance was being issued to NHS employers on the use of natural rubber latex in the NHS (Department of Health 2002). In 2003 a survey was conducted by the NPSA in conjunction with the Latex Allergy Support Group and the National Association of Theatre Nurses to ascertain the provision by the NHS for patients and staff who are allergic to latex in healthcare products (www.npsa.nhs.uk/latex/).

The Health and Safety Executive ordered the Great Western Hospital in Swindon to improve its systems for controlling exposure to latex after an employee suffered a serious allergic reaction. The hospital was given five months to plan how to minimise the risk to staff (*The Times* 2004).

In 2004 the Department of Health published guidance on a strategy for the risk assessment of chemical carcinogens (DoH 2004)

The HSE updated its guidance on latex in 2008 and on its website can be found answers to frequently asked questions on latex from both the employers' and employees' perspective. It states that the HSE policy is:

Single use, disposable natural rubber latex (NRL) gloves may be used where a risk assessment has identified them as necessary. When they are used they must be low-protein and powder-free.

The main findings of the risk assessment should be recorded. This will also help in instructing, informing and educating employees on the risks and appropriate control measures for natural rubber latex. Employers should put in place systems for ensuring that staff or patients with known latex allergies can work and be treated in a latex-safe environment.

Health surveillance and latex

As natural rubber latex is a potential asthmagen, health surveillance of staff is required. Single use disposable NRL gloves provide the majority of exposure to NRL.

As NRL produces a risk of asthma and dermatitis health surveillance is appropriate. The extent and detail of the health surveillance should be related to the degree of risk identified during the COSHH assessment and determined in consultation with an occupational health professional.

Health surveillance for non-powdered low protein gloves should include:

- An assessment of employees' respiratory health and skin condition, before they start a relevant job, to provide a baseline record.
- A regular (at least annual) enquiry for dermatitis and asthma. Such an enquiry might be undertaken by written questionnaire, orally during appraisal reviews, etc. Positive results should be referred to an occupational health professional for assessment.
- A responsible person identified and known to staff, competent to deliver these duties, and with lines of referral to an occupational doctor or nurse, for the reporting of symptoms as they might occur.
- For staff known to be sensitised to NRL and those considered to be at a high risk of developing sensitisation, i.e. atopic individuals, a higher level of health surveillance including a periodic clinical assessment by an occupational health doctor or nurse will normally be deemed appropriate.

The HSE website contains many case studies of health staff and others who suffered from latex reaction. In one case the mother of Nicola, aged 28, called her local ambulance service to treat Nicola's anaphylactic reaction to NRL in a consumer product (hair glue). The ambulance workers attempted to treat Nicola with standard resuscitation equipment but her symptoms worsened and she died. The ambulance service could not subsequently confirm that only latex-free equipment was used during resuscitation although plans were afoot to make latex-free packs available on all ambulances.

Health surveillance

The HSE has provided guidance on health surveillance by employers. It defines health surveillance as:

> *... any activity which involves obtaining information about employees' health and which helps protect employees from health risks at work.*

The objectives for health surveillance are:

- Protecting the health of employees by early detection of adverse changes or disease.
- Collecting data for detecting or evaluating health hazards.
- Evaluating control measures.

The HSE emphasises that health surveillance should not be confused with general health screening or health promotion. Health surveillance is necessary when:

- There is a disease associated with the substance in use (e.g. asthma, dermatitis, cancers).
- It is possible to detect the disease or adverse change and reduce the risk of further harm.
- The conditions in the workplace make it likely that the disease will appear.

Health surveillance is a process; it may be a regular planned assessment of one or more aspects of a worker's health, e.g. lung function or skin condition. However, it is not enough to simply carry out suitable tests, questionnaires or examinations. Employers must then have the results interpreted and take action to eliminate or further control exposure. It may be necessary to redeploy affected workers if necessary. Health surveillance may need to be completed by an occupational health service physician (doctor or nurse). If a GP offers the service, they must be competent in occupational medicine. The clinical outcomes from health surveillance are personal. The service provider must interpret the results of health surveillance for each individual and must supply general information for employees to keep up-to-date health records. Service providers may also be able to anonymise and group the information to highlight trends.

The HSE produces a priced publication called *Health Surveillance at Work* which provides guidance on how employers can fulfil their legal duty to provide health surveillance. The HSE also publishes *Understanding Health Surveillance at Work* (INDG304)

Self-employed persons

The COSHH regulations apply to those self-employed persons who are employers. The regulations (apart from those relating to monitoring and health surveillance) also apply if the self-employed person has no employees but takes substances to other people's premises.

New regulations

In 29 November 2010 the HSE gave information about two new European Regulations which were already having an impact on the way chemicals are supplied, packaged and labelled. The European Regulation (EC) No 1272/2008 on Classification, Labelling and Packaging of substances and mixtures (the CLP Regulation) came into force in all EU member states, including the UK, on 20 January 2010.

The CLP Regulation:

* Adopts in the EU the Globally Harmonised System (GHS) on the classification and labelling of chemicals.
* Is being phased in through a transitional period which runs until 1 June 2015. The CLP Regulation applies to substances from 1 December 2010, and to mixtures (preparations) from 1 June 2015.
* Applies directly in all EU member states. This means that no national legislation is needed.
* Is overseen by the European Chemicals Agency (ECHA).
* Will replace the Chemicals (Hazard Information and Packaging for Supply) Regulations 2009 (CHIP) from 1 June 2015.

Application of the law to *Scenario 10.1*

It is clear that there was a failure to ensure that the COSHH regulations were implemented in the children's ward at Roger Park Hospital. A straightforward risk assessment would have identified the dangers of bottles containing toxic substances being accessible to children who were not adequately supervised.

Measures should have been taken to ensure that children could not access such dangerous substances. To what extent is Daisy responsible? As ward manager she would have had the responsibility of ensuring that a COSHH assessment was undertaken, that the potential risks to the children on the ward were identified and that all reasonable measures were taken to ensure that they were not harmed. Even if she had been off duty at the time of the incident a failure to ensure that the risk assessment was carried out and implemented would be identified as her responsibility. Daisy would be professionally accountable for her actions: she could face prosecution under Section 7 of the Health and Safety At Work Act 1974 (see *Chapters 2 and 4*). Her failures could also be reported to the NMC. Her employer would be vicariously liable for any compensation due to the child. As a separate issue, there needs to be a policy on the supervision of children and the shared responsibility of parents and nursing staff.

Conclusion

The HSE has provided considerable help and guidance to assist in the implementation of the new 2002 COSHH regulations (as amended). Leaflets and videos and guidance are available from the HSE to assist employers and employees in fulfilling their statutory duties. The HSE also carried out a project in South Wales and asked major hazard sites to provide a list of their top 10 COSHH substances and work activities. The project focused on assessment and hazard identification, control, and monitoring. Further information is available on the HSE website.

Failure to comply with the regulations could lead to prosecution as well as civil action for compensation from employees and others who have suffered as a consequence of the failure to ensure that the substances hazardous to health are under appropriate control.

References

de Bruxelles S (2004) NHS must pay nurse £350,000 for allergy. *The Times* 17 June

Department of Health (2002) *Press Release 2002/0151. Guidance on the use of Latex in the NHS to be reissued.* DoH, London

Department of Health (2003) *Guidance on a Strategy for the Risk Assessment of Chemical Carcinogens.* DoH, London

Department of Health (2004) *Report of Committee on Carcinogenicity of Chemicals in Food, Consumer Products and the Environment.* DoH, London

Dugmore v. Swansea NHS Trust [2002] The Times 9 December CA

COSHH (2002) *The COSHH Regulations Statutory Instrument 2002 No 2677.* COSHH, London

Health and Safety Commission (2000) *Proposals for Reducing the Incidence of Occupational Asthma. CD164.* HSC, London

Health Services Executive (2000) *General Ventilation in the Workplace: Guidance for Employers.* HSE, London

Health Services Executive (2002) SI 2002/2677. Available from: www.hmso.gov.uk/si/si2002/2677.htm

Health Services Executive (2002 and updated) Preventing or Controlling Exposure to Hazardous Substances at Work. HSE, London. Available from: www. hse.gov.uk/hthdir/noframes/coshh/coshh9a.htm; www.hse.gov.uk/coshh/index.htm

Ogden v. Airedale Health Authority [1996] 7 Med LR 153

The Times (2004) News item Latex allergy. *The Times* 6 May

CHAPTER II

Medical devices

Scenario II.I. A medical device incident

Pansy suffered from a chronic lung condition which required frequent courses of antibiotics. As her veins were poor and cannulation was difficult, a passport was inserted into a vein in her arm in which antibiotics and other solutions were administered. After three courses of antibiotics over the course of several weeks, the nurses had difficulty in administering the medication through the passport but finally succeeded. Subsequently, during a routine X-ray of her lungs, it was discovered that the tube connected with the reservoir had become disconnected and had moved down the vein towards the heart.

Introduction

The Medical Devices Agency (MDA) was established in September 1994 as an executive arm of the Department of Health to promote the safe and effective use of devices. The Medical Devices Agency was subsequently incorporated (along with the Medicines Control Agency) into the Medicines and Healthcare Products Regulatory Agency (MHRA) which was set up in April 2003 (see below). In particular, the role of the MDA was to ensure that whenever a medical device is used, it is:

- Suitable for its intended purpose.
- Properly understood by the professional user.
- Maintained in a safe and reliable condition.

Its primary responsibility was to ensure that medical devices achieve the potential to help health care professionals give patients and other users the standard of care they have a right to expect. In order to fulfil this role it has six main functions:

- Investigating adverse incidents.
- Providing advice and guidance.

- Negotiating European directives and implementing and enforcing regulations on medical devices.
- Contributing to standard setting on medical devices.
- Evaluating medical devices and providing consultancy advice to users and purchasers.
- Providing support services for these activities.

Its website enables access to all its publications and notices (www.mhra.gov.uk).

What is a medical device?

The definition of a medical device used by the MDA is based upon the European Directive definition (European Union Directive 93/42/EEC) (*Box 11.1*) and incorporated into UK law by the 2002 Medical Devices Regulations (SI.2002/618).

'Medical device' means an instrument, apparatus, appliance, material or other article, whether used alone or in combination, together with any software necessary for its proper application, which

(a) is intended by the manufacturer to be used for human beings for the purpose of:

(i) diagnosis, prevention, monitoring, treatment or alleviation of disease,

(ii) diagnosis, monitoring, treatment, alleviation of or compensation for an injury or handicap,

(iii) investigation, replacement or modification of the anatomy or of a physiological process, or

(iv) control of conception; and

(b) does not achieve its principal intended action in or on the human body by pharmacological, immunological or metabolic means, even if it is assisted in its function by such means, and includes devices intended to administer a medicinal product or which incorporate as an integral part a substance which, if used separately, would be a medicinal product and which is liable to act upon the body with action ancillary to that of the device.

Medical devices regulations require that as from 14 June 1998 all medical devices placed on the market (made available for use or distribution even if no charge is made) must conform to 'the essential requirements' including

---

Box 11.1. Examples of medical devices

Annex B to Safety Notice 9801 from the MDA (1998a) gives examples of medical devices. See also the website: www.mhra.gov.uk. It covers the following:
- Equipment used in the diagnosis or treatment of disease, monitoring of patients, e.g. syringes and needles, dressings, catheters, beds, mattresses and covers, and other equipment
- Equipment used in life support, e.g. ventilators, defribillators
- Equipment used in the care of disabled people, e.g. orthotic and prosthetic appliances, wheelchairs and special support seating, patient hoists, walking aids, pressure care prevention equipment
- Aids to daily living, e.g. commodes, hearing aids, urine drainage systems, domiciliary oxygen therapy systems, incontinence pads, prescribable footwear
- Equipment used by ambulance services (but not the vehicles themselves), e.g. stretchers and trolleys, resuscitators
- Condoms, contact lenses and care products, intrauterine devices

---

safety required by law, and bear a CE marking as a sign of that conformity (SI 1994/3017, Directive 93/42/EEC).

Although most of the obligations contained in the regulations fall on manufacturers, purchasers who are positioned further down the supply chain may also be liable, e.g. for supplying equipment which does not bear a CE marking or which carries a marking liable to mislead people (MDA 1998b). This is the requirement of the EC Directive on medical devices (Directive 93/42/EEC). The manufacturer who can demonstrate conformity with the regulations is entitled to apply the CE marking to a medical device. The essential requirements include:

A device must not harm patients or users, and any risks must be outweighed by benefits.

(Directive 93/42/EEC)

Design and construction must be inherently safe, and if there are residual risks, users must be informed about them. Devices must perform as claimed, and not fail as a result of the stresses of normal use. Transport and storage must not have adverse effects. Essential requirements also include prerequisites in relation to design and construction, infection and microbial contamination, mechanical construction, measuring devices, exposure to radiation, built-in computer systems, electrical and electronic design, mechanical design, devices which deliver fluids to a patient, and function of controls and indicators. Exceptions to these regulations include the following:

- *In vitro* diagnostic devices (these are covered by separate regulations which came into force in 2000).
- Active implants (covered by the Active Implantable Medical Devices Regulations, Directive 90/385/EEC).
- Devices made specially for the individual patient ('custom made').
- Devices undergoing clinical investigation.
- Devices made by the organisation ('legal entity') using them.

In January 1998, the MDA issued a device bulletin (MDA 1998b) giving guidance to organisations on implementing the regulations. The MDA has powers under the Consumer Protection Act 1987 to issue warnings or remove devices from the market (*Chapter 12*).

Classification of devices

Devices are divided into three classes according to possible hazards, class 2 being further subdivided:

- Class 1 with a low risk, e.g. a bandage.
- Class 2a medium risk, e.g. a simple breast pump.
- Class 2b medium risk, e.g. a ventilator.
- Class 3 high risk, e.g. an intra-aortic balloon.

Any warning about equipment issued by the MDA should be acted upon immediately. Failure to ensure that these notices are obtained and acted upon could be used as evidence of failure to provide a reasonable standard of care.

Breast implants were subjected to stringent safety standards in Europe from 1 September 2003. The Department of Health had already classified that at the highest level of safety under the medical devices regulations.

Adverse incident reporting procedures

In 1998, the MDA issued a safety notice requiring health care managers, health care and social care professionals and other users of medical devices to establish a system to encourage the prompt reporting of adverse incidents relating to medical devices to the MDA (MDA 1998a). The procedures should be reviewed regularly, updated as necessary, and should ensure that adverse incident reports are submitted to the MDA in accordance with the notice.

What is an adverse incident?

The Safety Notice defines an adverse incident as 'an event which gives rise to, or has the potential to produce, unexpected or unwanted effects involving the safety of patients, users or other persons' (MDA 1998a). An adverse incident may be caused by shortcomings in:

> ... the device itself, instructions for use, servicing and maintenance, locally initiated modifications or adjustments, user practices including training, management procedures, the environment in which it is used or stored or incorrect prescription...

> (MDA 1998a)

where the incident has led to or could have led to the following:

> Death; life-threatening illness or injury; deterioration in health; temporary or permanent impairment of a body function or damage to a body structure; the necessity for medical or surgical intervention to prevent permanent impairment of a body function or permanent damage to a body structure; unreliable test results leading to inappropriate diagnosis or therapy.

> (MDA 1998a)

Minor faults or discrepancies should also be reported to the MDA (now the MHRA, see below).

Liaison officer

The Safety Notice suggests that organisations should appoint a liaison officer who would have the necessary authority to:

- Ensure that procedures are in place for the reporting of adverse incidents involving medical devices to the MDA.
- Act as the point of receipt for MDA publications.

- Ensure dissemination within their own organisation of MDA publications.
- Act as the contact point between the MDA and their organisation.

Medical Device Alert MDA/2011/01 (Device Bulletin DB 2010(01) *Reporting Adverse Incidents and Disseminating Medical Device Alerts*) gives advice to Medical Device Liaison Officers on their role in ensuring that comprehensive and effective systems are in place for the reporting of medical device-related adverse incidents to the MHRA and that these systems are regularly reviewed and maintained.

Guidance from the MHRA (incorporating the MDA)

The MHRA has published guidance on all aspects of the Medical Devices Regulations and the responsibilities of individuals and organisations (www.mhra. gov.uk). It has also published a checklist of questions for health professionals (*Box 11.2*) to ask themselves before they use medical devices (MDA 2001). An example of a warning issued by the MDA is that relating to a heart valve tester. It was reported that a 65-year-old woman died when her heart split in two after a heart valve tester broke when she was undergoing surgery. The MDA issued a hazard notice on 3 May 2002 warning about the specific tester (Teeman 2002). A list of all the publications of the MHRA setting out the title, the latest publication date, the

---

Box 11.2. Checklist for health professionals

- Do I know how to handle the medical devices in my unit?
- What preparation have I been given in how to use a medical device and was the preparation formalised and recorded or ad hoc?
- How was my competency to use this equipment safely assessed?
- Am I familiar with the instructions on how to use this piece of equipment and any warning labels?
- When was this equipment last serviced?
- Do my junior staff colleagues know how to use equipment?
- What is the cleaning and/or decontamination procedure and my responsibilities?
- Do I know who is responsible for risk management in my organisation?
- Do I know how to report an adverse incident?
- Do I know who my Medical Devices Agency liaison officer is?

Source: MDA (2001)

---

target audience, the type of guidance (regulatory, best practice, information) and the next review date, together with an internet link is available on the MHRA website.

One liners from the MHRA

One liners are adverse notices published by the MHRA on a regular basis to advise users of hazards. In June 2010 a special edition of one liners for dentists was published. In January 2011 the MHRA issued a collection of one liners specifically relating to maternity services especially for obstetricians and midwives. This included warnings about:

* The difference between UK and USA cardiotocograph (CTG) readers with different default settings for speed of the paper flow (in one case it was not realised after servicing that the main circuit board of the CTG had been replaced with the American default setting and an unnecessary emergency caesarean was performed).
* The CTG may record maternal heart rate not fetal heart rate. Even though the fetal scalp electrode was directly connected to the fetus, the fetus had died and the recording was a trace of the maternal heart rate.
* A baby crib from one manufacturer fell through its trolley base from a different manufacturer.
* An incorrectly placed umbilical cord clamp resulted in incomplete occlusion of the cord and led to severe neonatal blood loss.
* Automated blood pressure machines may give falsely low blood pressure readings when used for women with pre-eclampsia.
* Some birthing beds and babies' cots can tip, ejecting the occupant if the bed/cot is incorrectly loaded.

The MHRA advises that adverse incidents should be reported at the earliest opportunity. It prefers to receive reports via the online reporting system on its website. This online system may also be used to send an email copy of the report to the medical device liaison officer. The adverse incident hotline telephone number is 020 3080 7080. Detailed reporting guidance can be found on the MHRA website.

Needlestick injuries

The danger of staff receiving needlestick injuries is significantly high in health care. The concerns are so great that a seminar was held in March 2003 at the European

Parliament in Brussels on sharps injury prevention and single-use medical devices.

The announcement of the seminar stated that injuries caused by needles and other sharp medical devices and the related risk of potentially fatal disease transmission remain a major threat to the health and safety of health care workers across the European Union. In addition, the distress, sickness and absenteeism resulting from sharps injuries constitute a considerable strain on the already limited human resources in the medical profession. A Needle Stick Injury Bill which could have led to regulations being passed to prevent such injuries and to require statutory reporting of such incidents failed to complete its Parliamentary stages in 2003. Subsequently however initiatives within the European Community led to a directive (COM 2009 577) relating to the prevention of sharps injuries placing duties upon doctors, nurses and other health professionals including porters and cleaners to take action to prevent injuries. The directive gives legal effect to a framework agreement concluded by the European Hospital and Healthcare Employers' Association (HOSPEEM) and the European Federation of Public Service Unions (EPSU) through the social dialogue process which allows representatives of employers and workers to negotiate agreements on matters relating to employment and social affairs. The Directive came into force in June 2009 but three years were given for member states to prepare for compliance. The purpose of the Directive is to achieve the safest possible working environment by preventing injuries with all medical sharps including needlesticks; to protect workers at risk; to set up an integrated approach establishing policies in risk assessment, risk prevention, training, information awareness raising and monitoring and put in place response and follow-up procedures. At the heart of the Directive is the collaboration between employers and employees in the risk assessment of potential sharp hazards.

Medicines and Healthcare products Regulatory Agency (MHRA)

On 1 April 2003, the Medicines and Devices Agency merged with the Medicines Control Agency (MCA) to form the Medical Healthcare products Regulatory Agency (MHRA). The Department of Health considered that this merger would provide the opportunity to build on the undoubted strengths of the MCA and the new body would continue to be a world leader in terms of its scientific expertise and regulatory experience (Department of Health 2003). A report by the National Audit Office's (NAO's) 'Value for money' study which was published in January 2003, showed that the MCA had made a major contribution to the protection of public health through an efficient and effective licensing regime (NAO 2003).

An early alert from the new body related to venting systems on MRI scanners. This followed an incident in a Scottish Hospital where helium gas at minus 273°C, cold enough to freeze a patient to death, seeped into an examination room.

The future of the MHRA was considered in the review of arms' length bodies (Department of Health 2010) and the review concluded that as an Executive Agency of the Department of Health and a largely self-funding body through the fees it charges it did not propose to change its status nor to transfer its functions to another body.

Amendments to the Medical Devices Regulations

The current regulatory framework for medical devices has been in operation since 1998 with the regulations being amended in 2002 (The Medical Devices Regulations 2002 SI 2002/618). In 2005, a number of regulatory changes were proposed by the European Commission (EC) to strengthen the regime and improve implementation and thus better safeguard public health and maintain public trust and confidence in the regulatory framework. A revised Directive was agreed in 2007 (Directive 2007/47/EC) and was incorporated into UK law by the Medical Devices Amendment Regulations SI 2008 No 2936 which came into force on 21 March 2010. Some of the revisions simply clarify existing practice and are self-explanatory; other changes relate to the evaluation of clinical data. Where there is a lack of clinical data, manufacturers are required to justify this. Custom-made manufacturers are now required to review and document experience gained in the post-production phase and to set up a post-market surveillance system of reporting to authorities. Guidance has been prepared by the MHRA and is available on its website (www.mhra.gov.uk).

Overlap between Medical Devices Regulations and Personal Protective Equipment Regulations

Manufacturers are able to CE mark products dually as medical devices and personal protective equipment but are required to indicate which regulatory regime any products should come under or whether they come under both.

Flawed lens implants

In April 2004 it was reported that hundreds of patients who had undergone cataract operations had had a flawed lens implanted in their eyes and 304 patients needed a second operation to replace the lens (Hawkes 2004a). A Gloucester hospital had written to 1800 patients warning them about the lens and offering them the chance of seeing a specialist. A spokesman for the firm concerned said that the problem appeared to be the result of a reaction between the lens and a silicone gasket included in the packaging. The MHRA issued a warning on 5 April 2004 about another type of lens which had also caused clouding.

Single use items

The same European conference which considered the issue of injuries caused by needles and other sharp medical devices also considered the topic of the re-use of medical devices intended for single use. The conference briefing paper (www.eucomed.be) pointed out that the Medical Devices Directive (93/42/EEC) does not regulate the reprocessing of single use medical devices. The European Medical Technology Industry Association (Eucomed) is campaigning for the EU to regulate all reprocessing of medical devices intended for single use by medical practitioners, hospitals, reprocessors and original manufacturers in order to protect the health and safety of patients and health care workers. Its particular concerns on re-use of single use items relate to the general risk of infection and the risk of device impairment and to ensuring the consent of patients to the reuse.

The Medical Devices Agency issued guidance in 1995 (MDA 1995) on the re-use of single use items:

> *Medical devices on which the manufacturer has put the label 'single use' should not be re-processed and re-used unless the reprocessor is able to ensure the integrity and safety in use of each re-processed item; can produce documentary proof and evidence of successful validation studies of the re-processing operation; has a system for retaining full re-processing batch records, for subsequent retrieval in the event of a device failure and patient injury.*

The MDA pointed out that failure to comply with this guidance could result in the reprocessor becoming liable under the Consumer Protection legislation. (See *Chapter 12* and discussion on how the supplier can become liable instead of the manufacturer.)

Dangers with multiple use equipment

The Department of Health banned routine tonsil operations until they had the necessary disposable instruments. It was reported that parents were paying up to

£800 for surgical equipment to beat the ban (Charter 2001). In Wales tonsillectomy operations were halted in September 2002. The fear of infection from new variant Creutzfeldt-Jakob disease (CJD) meant that even re-usable instruments were considered to be safe for only one re-use. Tonsillectomies restarted in February 2003 on a phased basis with new disposable instruments.

Improvisation

In February 2004 the MHRA issued a warning that doctors and nurses should not use medical devices for purposes for which they are not intended (Hawkes 2004b). The MHRA gave examples of the death of two premature babies after wooden tongue depressors were used as splints to keep the arms of the babies in incubators still so they did not disturb the tubes inserted into them. The splints harboured a fungus which caused damage to blood vessels. Other examples included using a urinary catheter to tie a large wound closed, and using a wooden clothes peg to attach a device for measuring blood oxygen levels to an ear. The MHRA pointed out that many such adaptations had not passed scrutiny to ensure that they were safe. The report was criticised by a doctor in a letter to *The Times* (Ake 2004) on the grounds that nearly every new idea has come from some form of adaptation. However, any health professional should be aware that where equipment is adapted, the NHS trust may become the supplier for the purposes of liability under the Consumer Protection Act 1987 and this is considered in the next chapter.

Incentives and equipment

The Medicines (Advertising) Regulations 1994 stipulate that where relevant medicinal products are being promoted to persons qualified to prescribe or supply them, no person shall supply, offer or promise to such persons any gift, benefit in kind or pecuniary advantage. The National Audit Office warned in May 2004 that more than one-third of trusts had told the NAO that they had been offered incentives such as reduced prices to use new implants (Hawkes 2004c). One in 10 consultants are using hip implants for which there is inadequate evidence of effectiveness. The NAO suggested that the incentives may become an undue influence on purchasing decisions. They emphasised that incentives should be transparent and publicly declared and should not affect patient care. The NAO found that two thirds of incentives were not properly recorded and most free or subsidised international travel was not appropriately approved.

The MHRA reported on a complaint made by a pharmaceutical company against an incentive scheme involving insulin therapy. A pharmaceutical company complained in December 2004 about an incentive scheme offered to nurses involved in supporting the Sanofi-Aventis Insulin for Life (IFL) programme. This programme provided support for implementing health care and treatment for type 2 diabetes patients in primary care settings. The complainant was concerned that a direct financial reward paid to Ashfield Nurses for the number of patients started on insulin and indirect rewards for increasing the dose were prohibited, unethical and could compromise patient safety.

The complaint was not upheld because the Ashfield Nurses were not responsible for prescribing decisions and the scheme was designed to provide an incentive for successful training practices not the prescription of medicines. However, in the MHRA's opinion relating the remuneration given to individual nurses to the number of insulin starts made in the practices they support and for changes in dose was very ill-advised. Sanofi-Aventis responded that the incentive scheme was no longer running and that they would not be undertaking a similar exercise in the future. Full details of the scheme can be found on the MHRA website (Sanofi-Aventis Ashfield Nurses Incentive scheme for Insulin for Life programme).

Application of the law to *Scenario 11.1*

In relation to the situation in *Scenario 11.1* it is essential that as soon as it is found that the possibility of such a separation between the tubing and the reservoir could take place, a report must be sent to the MHRA. It should be clear within the NHS trust who has the responsibility of informing the liaison officer of the defect, so that the MHRA can warn the manufacturers and all users of this particular equipment of the danger. The MHRA has issued a leaflet on reporting faulty medical equipment giving contact details and identifying some of the ways in which it can go wrong (www.mhra.gov.uk). On the facts it does not appear that Pansy has suffered any direct harm, although there may have been increased discomfort during the administration of medicines. Fortunately, the defect was discovered before serious harm occurred. If Pansy had died as a result of the defect, her relatives may have had a claim under the consumer protection legislation, which will be considered in the next chapter.

Conclusion

The checklist provided by the MHRA is a useful starting point for any health professional not familiar with the Medical Devices Regulations. Assistance can be obtained within an NHS or primary care trust by contacting the MHRA liaison officer. At the very least, practitioners should ensure that they are on the circulation list for any relevant warnings from the MHRA and that they, in turn, know how to make known to the appropriate person an adverse incident should it arise. Personal access to the MHRA website would also ensure that practitioners keep up to date. At the heart of the safety of equipment is risk assessment and management, as the discussion on the sharps injuries and re-use of single use items illustrates. Other legislation such as the Consumer Protection Act 1987 relate to the safety of products and equipment and it is to this we turn in the next chapter.

References

Ake C (2004) Letter to the editor. *The Times* 10 February

Charter D (2001) Parents pay to beat ban on removal of tonsils. *The Times* 27 February

Department of Health (2003) *Medicines Control Agency. Press Release No. 2003/0018.* DoH, London: 15 January

Department of Health (2010) *Liberating the NHS: Report of the Arm's Length Bodies* D0H, London

Hawkes N (2004a) Cataract patients given flawed lens implants. *The Times*, 6 April

Hawkes N (2004b) Agency warns doctors not to improvise. *The Times* 5 February

Hawkes N (2004c) Doctors 'accept trips' for unproven hips. *The Times* 5 May

Medical Devices Agency (1995) *The re-use of medical devices supplied for single-use only.* MDA, London

Medical Devices Agency (1998a) *SN 90: Reporting Adverse Incidents Relating to Medical Devices.* MDA, London

Medical Devices Agency (1998b) *Medical Device and Equipment Management for Hospital and Community-based Organizations.* MDA DB 9801. MDA, London

Medical Devices Agency (2001) *One Liners* (Issue 11). MDA, London

National Audit Office (2003) *Value for Money* NAO London

Teeman T (2002) Heart-valve tester ban after death. *The Times* 4 May

Medicines and Healthcare products Regulatory Agency: 151 Buckingham Palace Road, London SW1W 9SZ. Telephone: 020 3080 6000 or contact them via their website: www. mhra.gov.uk

CHAPTER 12

Consumer protection

Scenario 12.1. A broken needle

Primrose is a doctor on a surgical ward. On one shift she was injecting Dora, a patient, with a painkiller when the needle broke, and the top part became embedded in Dora's arm.

Introduction

This chapter looks at the provisions of the Consumer Protection Act 1987 in relation to health care and the importance of retaining information about equipment and other products supplied to patients. The rights of the consumer to claim compensation when injured by defects in products were strengthened in 1987 by the Consumer Protection Act which was enacted as a result of the European Community Directive no. 85/37/374/EEC. Part 1 of the Consumer Protection Act 1987 makes provision for product liability and covers the sections shown in *Box 12.1*.

Box 12.1. Provisions of Part 1 Consumer Protection Act 1987

- Purpose and construction of Part 1 (of the Consumer Protection Act 1987)
- Liability for defective products
- Meaning of defect
- Defences
- Damage giving rise to liability
- Application of certain enactments
- Prohibition on exclusions from liability
- Power to modify Part 1
- Applications of Part 1 to the Crown

Consumer Protection Act 1987

The Consumer Protection Act 1987 enables a claim to be brought where harm has occurred as a result of a defect in a product. It is a form of strict liability in that negligence by the supplier or manufacturer does not have to be established. The claimant will, however, have to show that there was a defect. A product is defined as meaning any goods or electricity and includes a product which is comprised in another product, whether by virtue of being a component part or raw material or otherwise.

Who is liable under the Consumer Protection Act 1987?

Section 2(1) of the Consumer Protection Act 1987 states that:

> *Where any damage is caused wholly or partly by a defect in a product, every person to whom subsection (2) below applies shall be liable for the damage.*

Section 2(2) sets out who is liable under the Consumer Protection Act 1987 and is shown in *Box 12.2*. Usually it will be the producer of the defective goods who will be held liable under the Act, but it will be noted from *Box 12.2* that where the producer cannot be traced or is unknown then the supplier of the defective goods could be held liable. This has major implications for health care.

Records of the supplier

The fact that the supplier could be held liable under the Act makes it essential for the NHS trust to keep records of the supplier of any goods (including both equipment and drugs) which it provides for the client. In the absence of it being able to cite the name and address of the supplier, the NHS trust may become the supplier of the goods and therefore have to defend an action alleging that there was a defect in the goods which caused harm. Harm includes both personal injury and death and loss or damage of property.

Where a health service organisation supplies equipment for use in the community then that organisation can become the supplier for the purposes of the Consumer Protection Act 1987. If harm results from a defect in the equipment the appropriate supplier must provide the client with the name and address of the firm

---

Box 12.2. Consumer Protection Act 1987: Who is liable?

The producer: Section 2(2) includes the following as being liable:
- The producer of the product
- Any person who by putting his name on the product or using a trade mark or other distinguishing mark has held himself out to be the producer of the product
- Any person who has imported the product into the EEC in the course of business
- The supplier

In addition to the persons set out under section 2(2), section 2(3) enables any person who has been the supplier of the product to the person who suffered the damage or to the producer, shall be liable for the damage, if:
- The person who suffered the damage requests the supplier to identify one or more of the persons who were producers (as set out above)
- That request is made within a reasonable period after the damage occurs and at a time when it is not reasonably practicable for the person making the request to identify all those persons, and
- The supplier fails, within a reasonable period after receiving the request, either to comply with the request or to identify the person who supplied the product to him

---

from which the equipment was obtained otherwise it will become itself liable for the defects. Records of the source of equipment are therefore essential in order that the client can be given this information.

What is meant by a defect?

Section 3 of the Consumer Protection Act 1987 provides that:

There is a defect in a product for the purposes of part 1 of the Act, if the safety of the product is not such as persons generally are entitled to expect; and for those purposes, 'safety', in relation to a product, shall include safety with respect to products comprised in that product and safety in the context of risks of damage to property, as well as in the context of risks of death or personal injury.

115

The phrase what 'persons generally are entitled to expect' is further defined as taking into account all the circumstances which are shown in *Box 12.3*.

Box 12.3. Circumstances to be taken into account in determining what persons in general are entitled to expect

- The manner in which, and purposes for which, the product has been marketed, its get-up, the use of any mark in relation to the product and any instructions for, or warnings with respect to, doing or refraining from doing anything with or in relation to the product
- What might reasonably be expected to be done with or in relation to the product, and
- The time when the product was supplied by its producer to another

---

Defences

Certain defences are available under Section 4 and are shown in *Box 12.4*. The most significant of the defences set out in *Box 12.4* is (e). This is colloquially known as 'state of the art', i.e. that the state of scientific and technical knowledge at the time the goods were supplied was not such that the producer of products of that kind might be expected to have discovered the defect.

What damage must the claimant establish?

Compensation is payable for death, personal injury or any loss of or damage to any property (including land) (Section 5(1)). The loss or damage shall be regarded as having occurred at the earliest time at which a person with an interest in the property had knowledge of the material facts about the loss or damage (Section 5(5)). Knowledge is further defined in Section 5(6) and (7). Material facts about any loss of or damage to any property are such facts about the loss or damage as would lead a reasonable person with an interest in the property to consider the loss or damage sufficiently serious to justify his instituting proceedings for damages against a defendant who did not dispute liability and was able to satisfy a judgment. Knowledge includes knowledge which he might reasonably have been expected to acquire:

- from facts observable or ascertainable by him; or

Box 12.4. Defences under Consumer Protection Act 1987

(a) That the defect is attributable to compliance with any requirement imposed by or under any enactment or with any community obligation, or

(b) That the person proceeded against did not at any time supply the product to another, or

(c) That the following conditions are satisfied, i.e.: (i) that the only supply of the product to another by the person proceeded against was otherwise than in the course of a business of that person; and (ii) that section 2(2) does not apply to that person or applies to him by virtue only of things done otherwise than with a view to profit, or

(d) That the defect did not exist in the product at the relevant time, or

(e) That the state of scientific and technical knowledge at the relevant time was not such that a producer of products of the same description as the product in question might be expected to have discovered the defect if it had existed in his products while they were under his control, or

(f) That the defect (i) constituted a defect in a product (the subsequent product) in which the product in question had been comprised, and (ii) was wholly attributable to the design of the subsequent product or to compliance by the producer of the product in question with instructions given by the producer of the subsequent product

---

• from facts ascertainable by him with the help of appropriate expert advice which it is reasonable for him to seek;

but a person shall not be taken by virtue of this subsection to have knowledge of a fact ascertainable by him only with the help of expert advice unless he has failed to take all reasonable steps to obtain (and, where appropriate, to act on) that advice.

Action under the Consumer Protection Act 1987 in the health services

There have been some examples of actions being brought under the Consumer Protection Act 1987 in health care cases (Dimond 1993). One (reported in March 1993) led to Simon Garratt being awarded £1400 against the manufacturers of a pair of surgical scissors which broke during an operation on his knee, with the blade being left embedded. A second operation was required to remove it. Had Simon Garratt relied upon the law of negligence to obtain compensation he would have had to show that the manufacturers were in breach of the duty of care which they owed to him. Under the Consumer Protection Act 1987 he had to show only the harm, the defect and the fact that the equipment was produced by the defendant. A report by the National Consumer Council in November 1995 recommended that consumers should be assisted in using their rights under this Act (National Consumer Council 1995).

In one case (*Piper v. JRI (Manufacturing) Ltd* [2006]) involving hospital treatment, a claimant brought an action against manufacturers of an artificial hip which sheared in two beneath the femoral head close to the radial base of the spigot region of the stern. A further operation was required which lead to less movement and mobility. At the trial it was agreed that the prosthesis fractured as a result of fatigue failure initiating from a defect in the titanium alloy from which it was made. The defendants argued that there was no defect in the product when it left them, and that the defect occurred at the time of implantation. The trial judge found in favour of the defendants. The claimant's appeal failed.

The meaning of 'defect' in the Consumer Protection Act was considered by the Court of Appeal in a case brought against Tesco Stores (*Tesco Stores Ltd and another v. CFP (a minor by his litigation friend) and LAP* [2006]). In this case the trial judge had found Tesco and the manufacturer of the bottle to be in breach of the Consumer Protection Act in that the fitting on a bottle of dishwasher powder was not child proof. The mother had left her child of 13 months whilst she went to answer the phone and found the child sitting in the kitchen with the powder on his lips and his head right back. The mother was not found to be negligent. The Court of Appeal unanimously held that the definition of defect in the Act as 'if the safety of the product is not such as persons generally are entitled to expect' could not be interpreted to imply that every producer of a product warrants that the product fulfils its design standards. The public would expect that the bottle was more difficult to open than an ordinary screw top, although not so difficult as if the British Standard had been met. A requirement to meet British Standards could not be read into the Consumer Protection Act. There was therefore no breach of the Act.

In contrast in another case (*Abouzaid v. Mothercare (UK) Ltd* [2006]) brought under the Consumer Protection Act and the common law of negligence the Court of Appeal unanimously dismissed an appeal against an award of damages of almost £40 000 to a boy who at 12 years old was injured in the eye by the buckle on elastic straps attached to Cosytoes, a fleece-lined sleeping bag, which he was helping his mother attach to a pushchair. He lost the central vision of his left eye. The Court of Appeal held that there was a defect in the product because of the risk of the elasticated strap springing back into the eye. The defendant's argument that at the time the scientific and technical knowledge of the defect was not available did not succeed. The safety of the product was not such as persons generally are entitled to expect. There was however no finding of negligence at common law (see below).

In a claim for damages in relation to a defect in vaccination, the Court of Appeal unanimously dismissed an appeal against the trial judge's permitting the substitution of SmithKline Beecham in place of Merck as defendant even after the expiry of 10 years referred to in Section 11A(3) of the Limitation Act 1980 (*SmithKline Beecham v. Horne-Roberts* [2001]).

Blood products

In a case in 2001 (*A and Others v. National Blood Authority and Another* 2001) patients who had contracted hepatitis C from blood and blood products used in blood transfusions were able to succeed in a claim brought under the Consumer Protection Act 1987. Since the claimant does not have to establish under the Consumer Protection Act 1987 that there was negligence by the producer or supplier, the success of the patients who contracted hepatitis may well lead to greater use of the Consumer Protection Act 1987 in situations where personal injuries are caused as a result of defective products.

Compensation to haemophiliacs and others with hepatitis C

In August 2003 the Secretary of State for health announced that the Government intended providing compensation to those people who were infected with hepatitis C from contaminated blood products. A fund of £100 million was being set up for compensation and it is thought that sufferers would obtain between £20000 and £40000. The details of the scheme and payments were announced in January 2004 (Department of Health 2004). Under the scheme an *ex gratia* payment of up to £45000 would be payable to those who were alive on 29 August 2003 and whose hepatitis C infection is found attributable to NHS treatment with blood or blood products before September 1991. Those people infected will receive an initial lump sum payment of £20000 and those developing a more advanced stage of the illness, such as cirrhosis or liver cancer, will get a further £25000 and people who contracted hepatitis C through someone infected with the disease will also qualify for payment. The scheme was criticised by some because it excluded widows and those who had already died from the disease (Lister 2004). The Skipton Fund handles claims brought by those who have received contaminated blood (www.skiptonfund.org/Eng). An inquiry into the circumstances surrounding the supply to patients of contaminated blood and blood products was established under the chairmanship of Lord Archer of Sandwell to look at the consequences to the haemophilia community and others afflicted and suggest further steps to address their needs. Lord Archer's report was published in February 2009 and the Government published its response in May 2009 (Department of Health 2009). At the time of writing a Bill is being debated in Parliament which would, if passed, provide support for people who have been infected with certain diseases as a result of receiving contaminated blood and blood products supplied by the National Health Service. The Bill would establish a compensation package for people who have been infected, their widows, dependants and carers. It would also set up a committee to advise on the treatment of haemophilia and a review into the support available for infected people and their families (see *Chapter 24* for further details).

Action for negligence

Where a patient or other person has been injured as a result of defective equipment as well as being able to bring an action under the Consumer Protection Act 1987, he or she could also bring an action in the civil courts for negligence. In 1933 it was established in the famous 'snail in the ginger beer' case that the manufacturer owed a duty of care to the ultimate consumer even where the consumer had not personally paid for the goods and therefore had no contract with the supplier. The duty of care was owed in the law of negligence (*Donaghue v. Stevenson* [1932]). In an action for negligence, the injured person (or if the person has died, his or her personal representatives) must establish that a duty of care was owed, that there has been a breach of that duty by a failure to follow a reasonable standard of care (the Bolam Test is used to determine whether there has been such a failure (*Bolam v. Friern Barnet HMC* [1957]) and that this breach of duty caused the harm which the claimant has suffered. In contrast to an action brought under the Consumer Protection Act 1987 in an action for negligence, fault needs to be established and this is a significant hurdle for many claimants. The distinction is illustrated by the following case.

The Court of Appeal held that in deciding whether a product was defective in breach of Section 3 of the Consumer Protection Act 1987 (*Abouzaid v. Mothercare (UK) Ltd* [2000]) it was irrelevant whether the hazard had come, or ought reasonably to have come to the attention of the producer before the accident occurred. An absence of previous comparable accidents was however a relevant factor when deciding whether there had been a breach of the duty in negligence. In the case the claimant had suffered an eye injury as a result of the recoil of an elasticated strap attached to one of Mothercare's products. The Court of Appeal held that the product was defective within the meaning of the 1987 Act (and Article 6 of the Product Liability Directive (85/374/EEC)(OJ No 1985) but that there was no breach of the duty of care in negligence at common law. (For the law of negligence see *Chapter 5*. See above.)

Employers' Liability (Defective Equipment) Act 1969

Under this 1969 Act where an employee has been injured as a result of equipment provided by a third person, the injured employee can obtain compensation from the employer. The differences between an injured employee claiming compensation under the Consumer Protection Act 1987 in comparison with a claim under the Employers' Liability (Defective Equipment) Act 1969 is as follows:

- The injured employee can obtain compensation from the employer under the 1969 Act only if there has been negligence by a third party.
- The injured employee can obtain compensation from the employer as supplier only if he has not identified the producer under the 1987 Act.
- The 1987 Act covers all persons suffering damage, i.e. patients, employees, visitors, etc. The 1969 Act only relates to employees.
- The 1987 Act covers damages in the form of personal injury, death, loss or damage to property; the 1969 Act only covers loss of life, impairment of a person's physical or mental condition and any disease, not loss or damage to property.
- Fault need not be established under the 1987 Act – only a defect in the product. However, the defence of what is known at the time is available.

Contractual remedies and other statutory remedies

Where there is a contractual relationship between the parties or where the Sale of Goods and Services legislation applies, then other legal remedies would be available to the injured person. However, within the NHS the patient does not have a contract with the supplier of the equipment and therefore would rely on the law of negligence (if fault can be proved) or the Consumer Protection Act 1987. In contrast an employee does have a contract of employment and could therefore rely upon breach of the contract of employment in obtaining compensation from the employer.

Application of the law to *Scenario 12.1*

Dora would be able to claim under the Consumer Protection Act for harm resulting from the needle breaking. The trust would have to give her details of the producer, otherwise they could be liable as a supplier. Dora would have to show there was a defect in the needle and the fact she suffered harm. If there is evidence of any negligence by the doctor which caused the harm, the trust could be vicariously liable for the negligence.

Conclusions

It is possible that following the successful action by those patients who had contracted hepatitis C from blood and blood products used in blood transfusions that the Consumer Protection Act 1987 will be used more frequently when claims arise from defects in equipment. This applies not only to patients who are harmed by defective equipment but also to employees. The possibility of an increase in litigation using the Consumer Protection Act 1987 places more pressure on the need to ensure high standards of record keeping relating to the supply of equipment.

References

A and Others v. National Blood Authority and Another (2001) The Times Law Report 4 April 2001

Abouzaid v. Mothercare (UK) Ltd [2000] EWCA Civ 348

Bolam v. Friern Barnet HMC [1957] 1 WLR 582

Department of Health (2004) *Details of Hepatitis C ex-gratia payment scheme announced. Press release 2004/0025.* Department of Health, London

Department of Health (2009) *Government's response to Lord Archer's independent report on NHS supplied contaminated blood and blood products.* Stationery Office, London

Dimond BC (1993) Protecting the consumer. *Nursing Standard* 7(24): 18–19

Donaghue v. Stevenson [1932] AC 562

Lister S (2004) NHS hepatitis victims to get up to £45,000. *The Times*: 24 January

National Consumer Council (1995) *Unsafe Products. How the Consumer Protection Act Works for Consumers*. National Consumer Council, London

Piper v. JRI (Manufacturing) Ltd [2006] EWCA Civ 1344

Smithkline Beecham v. Horne Roberts [2001] EWCA Civ 2006

Tesco Stores Ltd and another v. CFP (a minor by his litigation friend) and LAP [2006] EWCA Civ 393

CHAPTER 13

National Patient Safety Agency

Scenario 13.1. Repetition of dangerous practices

May, the ward sister of an acute medical ward, was devastated when a young girl suffering from leukaemia died because an injection was given by a junior doctor as an epidural rather than into a vein. May subsequently heard that the same error had occurred several times before in the NHS, with fatal results. In her interview with the investigation team which was set up following the incident she deplored the fact that so many patients should die before the lessons were learnt.

Introduction

There are probably as many as 850 000 adverse health care events which occur each year in the NHS hospital sector. The financial costs of adverse events to the NHS is difficult to estimate, but are undoubtedly major and probably exceed £2 billion a year. One example of persistent failure to learn lessons is spinal injections. At least 13 patients have died or been paralysed since 1985 because a drug has been wrongly administered by spinal injection (Department of Health 2000a). This has led to revised guidance on intrathecal chemotherapy (see below).

An Organization with a Memory

The fact that the NHS failed to learn from repeated errors were the findings of the report *An Organization with a Memory* (Department of Health 2000a), written by an expert group chaired by Professor Liam Donaldson, Chief Medical Officer. The report put forward radical recommendations so that the situation in *Scenario 13.1* would not reoccur. The recommendations of the report included the points listed in *Box 13.1*.

Box 13.1. Recommendations of *An Organization with a Memory*

- The introduction of a mandatory reporting scheme for adverse health care events and 'near misses' based on sound, standardised reporting systems and clear definitions
- The introduction of a single overall database for analysing and sharing lessons from incidents and near misses, as well as litigation and complaints data which will identify common factors and consider specific action necessary to reduce risks to patients in the future
- The encouragement of a reporting and questioning culture in the NHS which moves away from 'blame' and encourages a proper understanding of the underlying causes of failures
- Improving NHS investigations and inquiries and ensuring that their results are fed into the national database so the whole NHS can learn lessons

Source: Department of Health (2000a)

Government response

The then Health Secretary Alan Milburn (Department of Health 2000b) gave strong support for the recommendations of the report, and authorised the Chief Medical Officer to implement the recommendations immediately with the aim of establishing a new national reporting system before the end of 2000. The aim of the new NHS national mandatory reporting system would be to log all adverse health incidents.

Target setting to reduce adverse health care events

An Organization with a Memory also recommended that the Department of Health should examine the feasibility of setting specific targets for the NHS to achieve in reducing the levels of frequently reported incidents (*Box 13.2*).

National Patient Safety Agency

In April 2001, the Department of Health published its proposals for establishing a National Patient Safety Agency to run the mandatory reporting system for logging all failures, mistakes, errors and near misses across the health services (Department

---

Box 13.2. Targets to reduce adverse health care events

- By 2001 reduce to zero the number of patients dying or being paralysed by wrongly administered spinal injections
- By 2005 reduce by 25% the number of instances of negligent harm in the field of obstetrics and gynaecology which result in litigation (these cases at that time accounted for around half the annual NHS litigation bill)
- By 2005 reduce by 40% the number of serious errors in the use of prescribed drugs (these at that time accounted for 20% of all clinical negligence litigation)
- By 2005 reduce to zero the number of suicides by mental health inpatients as a result of hanging from non-collapsible bed or shower curtain rails on wards (hanging from these structures was at that time the most common method of suicide on mental health inpatient wards)

---

of Health 2001a). The Department of Health's publication *Building a Safer NHS for Patients* (2001b) set out details of the scheme, together with recommendations for an improved system for handling investigations and inquiries across the NHS. It retained the targets set out by the report *An Organization with a Memory*.

The National Patient Safety Agency (NPSA) is an independent body which has the functions listed in *Box 13.3*. It was established as a special health authority under section 11 of the NHS Act 1977. Initially, it was to have between 12 and 15 non-officer members but this was changed by an amendment order to between

---

Box 13.3. Functions of the NPSA

- Collecting and analysing information on adverse events from local NHS organisations, NHS staff and patients and carers
- Assimilating other safety-related information from a variety of existing reporting systems and other sources in this country and abroad
- Learning lessons and ensuring that they are fed back into practice, service organisation and delivery
- Producing solutions to prevent harm where risks are identified
- Setting out national goals and establishing ways of tracking progress towards these goals

---

eight and 11, which also increased the officer members (apart from the Chief Executive) to three rather than one (National Patient Safety Agency (Establishment and Constitution) Order 2001 and Amendment Order 2003). The aim of this new national reporting system was to ensure that adverse events, including specified near misses, would be identified, recorded, analysed, and reported, and that lessons learnt would be shared to effect change at local and national levels. The NPSA coordinates its work with other reporting systems, e.g. RIDDOR (Reporting of Injuries, Diseases and Dangerous Occurrences) (*Chapter 14*), the Medical Devices Agency (MDA), and the Medicines Control Agency (MCA) which monitors adverse reactions to medicines. The MDA and the MCA have since been combined in a single organisation, the Medicines and Healthcare Products Regulatory Agency (MHRA) which commenced in April 2003 (*Chapter 11*).

The first chairman of the NPSA was Professor Rory Shaw, Medical Director of Hammersmith Hospital, appointed in August 2001 and he was succeeded by Lord Hunt in 2003. Flow charts showing how the scheme would work were set out in Chapter 3 of *Building a Safer NHS for Patients* (Department of Health 2001b).

Implementation timetable

Building a Safer NHS for Patients envisaged the following timetable:

- July 2001: Establishment of the NPSA.
- August 2001: Guidance to be provided on identifying and recording adverse events and near misses, with information being given to NHS organisations and staff.
- October 2001: Publication of a strategy for learning lessons.
- November 2001: Guidance to patients and carers on adverse events and how to report them.
- December 2001: 60 percent of NHS trusts will be able to provide information to the national system
- December 2002: All NHS trusts to be providing information.

Minimum data set for adverse event and near-miss reporting

Documentation for reporting requirements should include the following information:

- What happened?
- Where did it happen?
- When did it happen?
- How did it happen?
- Why did it happen?
- What action was taken or proposed?
- What impact did the event have?
- What factors did, or could have, minimised the impact of the event?

Barriers to reporting

The report recognised that there are many barriers which will have to be overcome in any reporting system. These are identified as follows:

- Lack of awareness of the need to report, what to report and why.
- Lack of understanding of how to report.
- Staff feel that they are too busy to make a report.
- Too much paperwork involved in reporting.
- Patient recovers from the adverse event and the urgency goes out of the situation.
- Fear of point-scoring by colleagues, retribution by line management, disciplinary action or litigation.
- An assumption that someone else will make the report.
- No evidence of timely feedback and/or corrective action being taken resulting from making a report.

It is the task of the NPSA to provide guidance on how these barriers can be removed.

Internal inquiries

The report recommended that in future, instead of an internal inquiry following a major service failure, after notification to the regional office of the Department of Health, the Department of Health and Commission for Health Improvement (from April 2004 the Commission for Healthcare Audit and Inspection and from 2009 the Care Quality Commission) would determine the appropriate form of investigation. This would possibly be an independent external investigation or inquiry or, in exceptional circumstances, a Secretary of State inquiry under his statutory powers.

Complaints from staff

It was envisaged that the core of the new adverse event system would be reports made by NHS staff. Chapter 2 of *Building a Safer NHS for Patients* stated that:

> *The success will depend on creating an open culture within all NHS organisations where staff feel that they can draw attention to errors or mistakes (so that learning can take place) without fear of disciplinary action. A confidential channel will also be created for reporting.*

> (Department of Health 2001b)

Research into safety

Included in the proposals was a discussion on the key questions to be answered in developing a patient safety research agenda. The Department of Health has commissioned research to establish: the size and nature of the problem; understanding the factors which cause harm and assessing the efficacy of intervention strategies; developing and designing reporting systems to help ensure their good use; learning lessons and disseminating them; changing individual and organisation behaviour; and involving patients.

It was envisaged that the NPSA would take the lead in strengthening the relationship between the various bodies funding research into patient safety. Clinical specialist advisers to the NPSA are appointed jointly by the NPSA and the Royal Colleges. They provide advice to the NPSA on practical solutions to safety issues.

First annual report of the NPSA

In the first six months of its work, the NPSA, in association with other bodies such as NICE, MDA, and MCA, pharmacists, and NHS trusts, covered the following topics:

- The carrying of antidote naloxone by ambulance teams.
- Safety measures to prevent overdose of potassium chloride.
- Antibiotic coated catheters.
- Breathing equipment in theatres.
- Infusion pump user issues.

One of the key objectives of the NPSA is to assist in the development of a climate within the health service in which open reporting and learning can take place. To support this process it has set up stakeholder workshops, undertaken research into public perceptions of risk in relation to health and worked with the Department of Health Personnel Directorate on aspects of the national human resources agenda to achieve this cultural change.

The National Patient Safety Agency annual report for 2002 covering 2001–2002 in December 2002 (NPSA 2002a) also indicated the ways in which it was establishing the service. Twenty-eight pilot schemes had been set up and were evaluated in an extensive report (NPSA 2002c). The pilots tested how the system:

- Records, codes information and classifies data.
- Links recording and analysis of data with other appropriate information.
- Learns lessons from the analysis.

The conclusions of the evaluation report have lead to improvements in the IT system so that an efficient and effective rollout of a national reporting system has been implemented. It has also assisted in determining how to manage the large volumes of data and define who is responsible for data quality. Recommendations were also made on the need to develop a patient safety culture in the NHS and the need to support the NHS by developing guidance on classification of incidents and near misses, and incident reporting. The latter recommendation required establishing comprehensive training and development strategies to ensure that the NPSA supports and facilitates trusts' initiatives. It is evident from the evaluation report that the NPSA has faced and still faces an enormous challenge in changing the climate in the NHS so that staff are prepared to report adverse incidents and are not inhibited by the fear of repercussions.

The NPSA's first patient safety alert was issued on 23 July 2002 and was about preventing accidental overdose with intravenous potassium (NPSA 2002b). The alert notice refers to the possible risks from treatment with concentrated potassium and the need for additional safety precautions in the way potassium solutions are stored and prepared in hospital. The alert on potassium chloride was updated in 2003. The NPSA co-operated with the Design Council to examine how the effective use of design can reduce the risk of medical error. An example can be seen in preventing drugs being given epidurally when they are intended for intravenous administration. (For the NPSA and infection control see *Chapter 15*.)

Seven Steps to Patient Safety

The NPSA published in November 2003 (reprinted 2004) *Seven Steps to Patient Safety* in order to ensure the creation of a safety culture and the appropriate systems and processes (see NPSA website). These are shown in *Box 13.4*.

Primary care and the NPSA

In May 2003 it was announced that GPs were to be included in the reporting scheme. Research had revealed that up to 2.8 million GP consultations every year result in a medical error (Wright 2003).

National Guidance on the Safe Administration of Intrathecal Chemotherapy

The Department of Health issued updated *National Guidance on the Safe Administration of Intrathecal Chemotherapy* in 2003 (Department of Health 2003b). NHS trusts were required to be fully compliant with the guidance contained in the Annex to the circular by 30 November 2003. A training toolkit

---

Box 13.4. *Seven Steps to Patient Safety*

- Step 1. Build a safety culture – create a culture that is open and fair
- Step 2. Lead and support your staff – establish a clear and strong focus on patient safety throughout your organisation
- Step 3. Integrate your risk management activity – develop systems and processes to manage your risks and identify and assess things that could go wrong
- Step 4. Promote reporting – ensure your staff can easily report incidents locally and nationally
- Step 5. Involve and communicate with patients and the public – develop ways to communicate openly with and listen to patients
- Step 6. Learn and share safety lessons – encourage staff to use root cause analysis to learn how and why incidents happen
- Step 7. Implement solutions to prevent harm – embed lessons through changes to practice, processes or systems

---

and video were issued to support local induction and training programmes. The Chief Executive of each NHS trust is required to identify a designated lead to oversee compliance within the trust. Trusts that undertake less than 10 procedures a year (low volume trusts) should carry out a risk assessment to decide if they should continue to provide the service at all. High level trusts (500+ procedures per annum) should carry out a risk assessment to check the capacity and safety of the service, a written local protocol should be drawn up and a register established to identify personnel who have been trained and are authorised to prescribe, dispense, issue, check or administer; automatic inclusion in a hospital's register on the transfer of staff should not occur. There should be annual reviews of competence and a certificate or other written confirmation of competence should be issued. The guidance also includes advice on those eligible to prescribe, and on documentation, storage, and administration of intrathecal chemotherapy. After intravenous chemotherapy has been administered, an area should be designated for the administration of intrathecal chemotherapy and it should only be administered in normal working hours. Guidance on waivers is also given.

NPSA guidance on safer use of infusion devices

On 24 May 2004 the NPSA released new guidelines to promote safer use of infusion devices used to release fluids and medication into a patient's body (www.npsa. nhs.uk/infusiondevices). The Safer Practice Notice outlines the steps that hospitals can take to improve patient safety and make significant cost savings. The NPSA estimated that if a hospital reduced the number of infusion devices by 10 percent, it could save, on average, £120000 per year. Its package of solutions includes:

- An assessment to review existing infusion device purchasing processes and a checklist to help trusts ensure that the right people are involved in decision making.
- A questionnaire to help in the evaluation of devices prior to purchase.
- Advice for trusts on how to develop a business case for an equipment library or other centralisation facility.
- A spreadsheet to help trusts establish a local economic appraisal.

These solutions are available on its website (www.npsa.nhs.uk/infusiondevices). The NPSA has also worked to develop an accredited e-learning programme for all staff who use infusion devices, using a national competency framework which has been available since 2004.

Incident decision tree

In 2003, the National Audit Office reported that 1000 full-time clinical staff were excluded between April 2001 and July 2002 which cost the NHS an estimated £29 million (National Audit Office 2003).

A summary version of *Seven Steps to Patient Safety* is available on the NPSA website. The full guide includes the evidence for each step, practical tips, and details on NPSA resources of direct relevance to NHS staff.

The National Audit Office found that a number of staff were inappropriately suspended due to system failures rather than individual shortcomings. The NPSA has also developed a decision-making tool to help NHS managers decide whether to suspend staff facing allegations over patient safety. By cutting the number of inappropriate suspensions the move could save the health service millions of pounds a year. The incident decision tree (ICT) is an electronic, interactive system which, through a systematic series of questions, should assist managers in deciding if staff should be suspended or if there are alternatives to suspension such as a change of duties. Further details can be obtained on the NPSA website (www.npsa.nhs.uk/idt).

One crash call number

The NPSA announced in April 2004 that it was recommending that all NHS Acute Trusts across England and Wales should standardise to one crash call telephone number in a move to reduce confusion in emergencies and to improve patient safety. The number suggested was 2222.

National Reporting and Learning Service (NRLS)

The NRLS was developed by the NPSA and launched in February 2004 and was aimed at drawing together reports of patient safety errors and system failures from health professionals across England and Wales and to help the NHS to learn from things that go wrong. It has been designed to extract information from existing local risk management systems. This includes electronic reporting known as eForm. The system has been extended to the whole of England and Wales, and the NPSA publishes statistics on trends and issues identified through NRLS to promote a learning culture in the NHS. It provides feedback to NHS organisations and uses the data to prioritise the development of safety solutions from improved patient safety.

Alerts issued by the NRLS in recent months include:

- Safer spinal (intrathecal), epidural and regional devices (31 January 2011).
- Essential care after an inpatient fall (13 January 2011).
- Safer ambulatory syringe drivers (16 December 2010).
- Preventing fatalities from medication loading doses (25 November 2010).
- The transfusion of blood and blood components in an emergency (21 October 2010).
- Laparoscopic surgery: Failure to recognise post-operative deterioration (23 September 2010).
- Prevention of over-infusion of intravenous fluid and medicines in neonates (26 August 2010).
- Reducing treatment dose errors with low molecular weight heparins (30 July 2010).
- Safer administration of insulin (16 June 2010).
- Reducing the risk of retained swabs after vaginal birth and perineal suturing (26 May 2010).
- Checking pregnancy before surgery (28 April 2010).
- Early detection of complications after gastrostomy (31 March 2010).
- Reducing harm from omitted and delayed medicines in hospital (24 February 2010).
- Safer use of intravenous gentamicin for neonates (09 February 2010).
- Vaccine cold storage (21 January 2010).
- Reducing the risks of tourniquets left on after finger and toe surgery (09 December 2009).
- Safer lithium therapy (01 December 2009).
- Being open: communicating patient safety incidents with patients (19 November 2009).
- Oxygen safety in hospitals: Rapid Response Report (29 September 2009).
- Minimising risks of suprapubic catheter insertion (adults only) (29 July 2009).

Other initiatives of the NPSA included the launch in May 2010 of plans to reduce levels of harm in 10 high risk patient safety areas. The 10 high risk clinical areas were identified and the actions organisations needed to take to reduce them from re-occurring were set out.

In July 2010 the NPSA adopted a zero tolerance policy for pressure ulcers and was encouraging all NHS organisations to work towards complete prevention. The NPSA stated:

The solutions are very simple; observing patients' skin and changing the position of patients at regular intervals as well as checking for a moisture free environment and monitoring their nutritional status. These small changes should make a big difference to reduce the chances of pressure ulcers from developing. In addition, the NPSA will be conducting a number of briefings and workshops at NHS organisations, highlighting and urging staff to share best practice and to support local and national educational initiatives.

In January 2011 the NPSA issued guidance to NHS organisations in England and Wales, aimed at improving care after a patient has suffered a fall in a clinical setting. NHS organisations with inpatient beds are encouraged to ensure safe manual handling and prompt assessment and treatment of a patient after a fall has happened as this greatly increases the chances of a patient making a full recovery. Each year around 282 000 patient falls are reported to the NPSA. This latest Rapid Response Report (RRR) was produced because a proportion of the patients suffering injuries did not receive prompt and correct diagnosis and treatment of their injuries. A significant number of these result in death, or severe or moderate injury, including around 840 fractured hips, 550 other types of fracture and 30 intracranial injuries.

National recognition for the quality and clarity of NPSA reports

In September 2010 the NPSA was given national recognition for the quality and clarity of clinical information contained within its Rapid Response Reports. The NHS Evidence Accreditation Scheme – a national programme that recognises the high quality of information for health and social care staff – found that the NPSA has robust systems in place to produce the guidance. Assessors noted that the NPSA involved a wide range of stakeholders when producing each report and that the recommendations were clear and specific and were distributed widely and rapidly.

Failure of NHS to take action on alerts

In spite of the commendation of the NPSA for the clarity of its rapid response reports, in February 2011 the charity Action Against Medical Accidents (AvMA) published a report, *Implementation of Patient Safety Alerts: Too Little Too Late?* which took a snapshot of alerts that had not been acted upon from 2004 to 20 January 2011. A summary of its findings were:

- There were 654 instances of patient safety alerts which had not been complied with. Whilst this represents a decrease of 50 percent on the August 2010 figure, each alert not complied with means that lives are being put at unnecessary risk. All alerts are supposed to be complied with by all trusts by the given deadline, and trusts have been reminded of this requirement by the Department of Health.
- 203 (50 percent) trusts had failed to comply with at least one alert.
- 45 trusts had not complied with five or more alerts. Five trusts had not complied with 10 or more alerts.
- Many of the alerts which had not been complied with were years past the deadline for completion. For example, 'Safer use of Injectable Medicines' (deadline for completion 31 March 2008) had not been complied with by 26 trusts. 'Right Patient Right Blood' (deadline for completion 1 May 2009) had not been complied with by 36 trusts.
- Even extra urgent 'Rapid Response Alerts' had not been complied with by many trusts. For example, rapid response alert 'Oxygen Safety in Hospitals' (deadline for completion 29 March 2010) had not been complied with by 31 trusts.
- Some trusts which had been among the worst performers in the AvMA's last two reports and to whom the Care Quality Commission had been moved to write to to remind them of the need to comply, still have over 10 alerts outstanding. For example, Stockport NHS Foundation Trust had 14 alerts outstanding (15 in February 2010); Manchester PCT had 13 outstanding (23 in February 2010); Barts and the London NHS Trust had 11 alerts outstanding (20 in February 2010); and Aintree University Hospitals NHS Foundation Trust had 10 alerts outstanding (12 in February 2010).

The report included heart-rending case studies of patients who had died because alerts had not been implemented. The recommendations of the AvMA are:

- The Care Quality Commission should be more proactive in insisting with compliance with patient safety alerts and taking action with trusts who continue not to comply. Starting with the trusts with multiple alerts outstanding and those who are more than a year overdue with complying with an alert, trusts should be made to produce an action plan for complying within a short timescale or face sanctions.
- The Department of Health should produce a business plan for the co-ordination of patient safety work, including the generation of and

monitoring compliance with patient safety alerts. This should include detail on how this work will be co-ordinated when the new system is up and running and in the immediate short-term period of transition.

• Information on compliance with patient safety alerts should be made available in a far more prominent and user-friendly way than is the case presently. If patients and the public could readily see if trusts were complying or not on the trust's own website and through NHS Choices, this would provide a powerful incentive for trusts.

• There needs to be a concerted programme of training for NHS staff drawing on the best practice that has allowed 50 percent of trusts to comply with patient safety alerts and real patient stories demonstrating how vitally important this is.

Arms' length bodies review

In 2010 the Review of Arms' length bodies (Department of Health 2010) proposed the following future for the NPSA:

3.60 We propose to abolish the National Patient Safety Agency. Some National Patient Safety Agency functions will become part of the remit of the NHS Board, while others will be supported to continue in other ways. The following functions will transfer to elsewhere in the wider health system:

3.61 The work of the Patient Safety Division relating to reporting and learning from serious patient safety incidents should move to the NHS Commissioning Board, as a Patient Safety sub-committee of the Board, covering the whole function from getting evidence to working up evidence-based safe services. This would provide an opportunity to preserve the synergy between learning and operational practice that already exists in the system. We will engage with the National Patient Safety Agency to discuss the transitional arrangements for the Patient Safety Division.

3.62 The National Clinical Assessment Service, which helps health care managers and practitioners to understand, manage and prevent concerns with the performance of doctors, dentists and pharmacists, should continue in the short term. It is valued by employers of doctors, dentists and pharmacists whose performance calls for rehabilitation to ensure continued safe practice. However, there is an expectation that revalidation of the medical profession and other incentives in the system will reduce the need for this service in the future. We propose that, over the next few years, the National Clinical Assessment Service will become a self-funded service and the Department intends to agree a date with the service for achieving self-sufficiency.

3.63 The National Research Ethics Service helps protect the interests of patients and research participants in clinical trials and facilitates and promotes ethical research. It includes recognising and authorising Research Ethics Committees, which approve individual research applications. We propose that the future of the National Research Ethics Service is considered as part of the wider Academy of Medical Science's review of research regulation with a view to moving this function into a single research regulatory body.

3.64 The National Patient Safety Agency currently commissions three confidential enquiries to provide learning on what went wrong in adverse health care incidents. In future, the enquiries could sit with the National Clinical Audit Patient Outcome Programme (NCAPOP consists of 30 individual national clinical audits) managed on behalf of the Department by the Healthcare Quality Improvement Partnership (HQIP).

3.65 We will engage with the National Patient Safety Agency about the implementation of the proposals contained in this document.

At the time of writing these proposals are still to be implemented.

Applying the law to *Scenario 13.1*

Following the establishment of the NPSA there should be a reduction in the repetition of dangerous practices. May should obviously ensure that a report of the incident is made and the appropriate accident forms completed. The health and safety officer in the trust should ensure that the appropriate statutory notifications take place.

In a case similar to *Scenario 13.1* a doctor in Nottingham pleaded guilty to the manslaughter of a patient to whom he had administered vincristine by epidural rather than intravenously. He was given a prison sentence, but was released after sentencing because of the time he had spent remanded in custody. If the revised guidance on intrathecal chemotherapy issued by the Department of Health in 2003 is implemented, the target of zero intrathecal errors should be achieved.

Conclusions

As the barriers to reporting listed above show, the national scheme of reporting will only work if it has the support of staff. In order to achieve this support, the NPSA must prove that it can provide the information required without setting up more red tape and bureaucratic frustrations. The Department of Health published a consultation document *Making Amends* (Department of Health 2003a) which envisaged that a new statutory scheme for obtaining compensation for clinically significant changes would be established alongside the existing civil court procedure. As part of its recommendations it suggested that there should be legislation to create a duty on health care professionals and managers to inform patients where they become aware of a possible negligent action or omission. However, it recommended that this should be linked with provision for an exemption from disciplinary action by employees or professional regulatory bodies for those reporting adverse events except where the health care professional has committed a criminal offence or it would not be safe for the professional to continue to treat patients.

To provide further incentive to the reporting of adverse events it recommended that documents and information collected for identifying adverse events should be protected from disclosure in court. It recommended that this protection should only apply to reports of adverse events where full information on the event was also included in the medical record. The NHS Redress Act 2006, which followed this consultation document, has not yet been brought into force and at the present time seems unlikely ever to be so. The Report of the AvMA showing the low rate of NHS Trust implementing the NPSA alerts illustrates how far the NHS has to go in improving standards of health and safety. The Coalition Government is planning the abolition of the NPSA with its functions being transferred to other organisations. There is little guarantee that these changes will result in higher standards.

References

Department of Health (2000a) *An Organization with a Memory. Report of an expert group chaired by Professor Liam Donaldson*. DoH, London

Department of Health (2000b) *National System for NHS to Learn from Experience. 2000/349*. DoH, London

Department of Health (2001a) *National Patient Safety Agency to be launched. Press release*. DoH, London

Department of Health (2001b) *Building a Safer NHS for Patients*. DoH, London

Department of Health (2003a) *Making Amends. A consultation paper setting out proposals for reforming the approach to clinical negligence in the NHS*. CMO: June

Department of Health (2003b) *Updated National Guidance on the Safe Administration of Intrathecal Chemotherapy. HSC 2003/010*. DoH, London: October

Department of Health (2010) *Liberating the NHS: Report of the Arm's Length Bodies* London Crown

National Audit Office (2003) *The Management of Suspensions of Clinical Staff in NHS Hospital and Ambulance Trusts in England*. NAO, London

National Patient Safety Agency (2000) *Pilot Evaluation Report 22 May 2002*; www.npsa. nhs.uk/publications

National Patient Safety Agency (2002a) *Annual Report 2001–2002*. NPSA, London

National Patient Safety Agency (2002b) *Patient Safety Alert PSA 01*. NPSA, London

National Patient Safety Agency (2004) *Seven Steps to Patient Safety Full Reference Guide* NPSA

National Patient Safety Agency (Establishment and Constitution) Order 2001 S I 2001 No 1743 and Amendment Order 2003 S I 2003 No 1077

Wright O (2003) GPs will own up to errors in 'near miss' log. *The Times* 21 May

CHAPTER 14

Reporting of injuries, diseases and dangerous occurences (RIDDOR)

Scenario 14.1. An accident form

Clematis, an occupational therapist working in an orthopaedic ward, injured her back when lifting a patient with another health professional from the bed to a wheelchair. She was admitted to hospital and was off sick for many weeks. When she returned to work she noticed that the accident form which she had completed was still on the ward and copies did not appear to have been circulated. What is the law and what is her responsibility?

Introduction

The regulations which were introduced in 1985 governing the reporting of injuries, diseases and dangerous occurrences (RIDDOR), were replaced by new regulations which came into force on 1 April 1996 (Health and Safety Executive 2009). Guidance by the Health and Safety Executive (HSE), which was updated in 2009, sets out full details of the regulations, the schedules and appendices. (Further information explaining how RIDDOR works is available on www.hse. gov.uk.) There is now one set of regulations in place and the list of reportable diseases has been updated, as has the list of dangerous occurrences. It is now legally possible for reports to be made by telephone (see below). The Reporting of Injuries, Diseases and Dangerous Occurrences Regulations 1995 (RIDDOR), place a legal duty on:

- employers,
- self-employed people, and
- people in control of premises,

to report work-related deaths, major injuries or over-three-day injuries, work-related diseases, and dangerous occurrences (near miss accidents). The usual way to do this is by calling the Incident Contact Centre (ICC) on 0845 300 99 23 (local rate). A copy of the information recorded will be sent to the informer who will be able to correct any errors or omissions.

Following the successful HSE pilot scheme in Scotland, in February 2000 it was announced that funding was to be made available to the HSE to set up a centralised national workplace accident and incident reporting system instead of the 500 different addresses which were then in use (Health and Safety Executive 2000). Reports can be made to the HSE in the following ways:

* Telephone: 0845 300 9923.
* Internet: www.hse.gov.uk/riddor.
* E-mail: riddor@natbrit.com.
* Post: Incident Contact Centre Caerphilly Business Park, Caerphilly CF83 3GG

Box 14.1 shows the contents of the regulations.

Box 14.1. RIDDOR regulations

1. Citation and commencement
2. Interpretation
3. Notification and reporting or injuires and dangerous occurrences
4. Reporting of death of an employee
5. Reporting of cases of disease
6. Reporting of gas incidents
7. Records
8-10 Quarries, offshore workplaces and restrictions on the applications of the regulations
11. Defences

Schedules include:
1. Major injuries
2. Dangerous occurrences
3. Reportable diseases
4. Records

Appendices include:
1. Means of contacting HSE
2. Report forms
3. Certificates of exemption

Definitions

An 'accident' is defined as including:

- An act of non-consensual physical violence done to a person at work.
- An act of suicide which occurs on, or in the course of the operation of, a relevant transport system.

'Disease' includes a medical condition, and 'major injury' means an injury or condition which is specified in Schedule 1. These include:

- Any fracture, other than to the fingers, thumbs or toes.
- Any amputation.
- Dislocation of the shoulder, hip, knee or spine.
- Loss of sight (whether temporary or permanent).
- A chemical or hot metal burn to the eye or any penetrating injury to the eye.
- Any injury resulting from an electric shock leading to unconsciousness or requiring resuscitation or admittance to hospital for more than 24 hours.
- Any other injury leading to hypothermia, heat-induced illness or unconsciousness.
- Any condition requiring resuscitation or requiring admission to hospital for more than 24 hours.
- Loss of consciousness, caused by asphyxia or by exposure to a harmful substance or biological agent.
- Either of the following conditions which result from the absorption of any substance by inhalation, ingestion or through the skin: acute illness, requiring medical treatment or loss of consciousness.
- Acute illness which requires medical treatment where there is reason to believe that this resulted from exposure to a biological agent or its toxins or infected material.

Some of these terms are further defined. Schedule 3 sets out the occupational diseases which come under the reporting regulations. They are divided between those conditions which are the result of physical agents and the physical demands of work (such as carpal tunnel syndrome), infections as a result of biological agents (such as hepatitis), and conditions resulting from substances (such as bladder cancer, occupational dermatitis and occupational asthma).

Requirements of the regulations

If a death, major injury or injury requiring hospital admission or a dangerous incident (as defined in Schedule 2) occurs, then regulation 3 requires the responsible person:

- To notify 'forthwith' the relevant enforcing authority by the quickest practicable means.
- To send, within 10 days, a report thereof to the relevant enforcing authority on an approved form or format.

This regulation also applies if a person who is not at work is injured on hospital premises as a result of an accident arising out of or in connection with work. This ensures that accidents at hospitals are also reported. In addition, reports should be made where employees are injured at work and are off work or unable to do their normal duties for more than three consecutive days.

Exclusion of injury under medical supervision

Under regulation 10, the reporting requirement does not apply to the death or injury of a person arising out of the conduct of any operation on, or any examination or other medical treatment of, that person which is administered by, or conducted under the supervision of, a registered medical practitioner or a registered dentist. The guidance explains that this exclusion does not apply to injuries arising from accidents to patients occurring under any other circumstances. It gives the example of a patient dying or suffering a major injury as a result of a power failure during an operation (and not caused by the conduct of the operation). The death or major injury must be reported.

Records

The employer is required to keep a record of:

- Any event which is required to be reported under regulation 3 and this shall contain the particulars specified in part 1 of schedule 4.
- Any case of disease required to be reported under regulation 5(1) and this shall contain the particulars specified in part 2 of schedule 4.
- Such other particulars as may be approved by the executive for the purpose

of demonstrating that any approved means of reporting under regulations 3 or 5(1) have been complied with.

These records must be kept for three years and records kept for other purposes will satisfy the requirements of regulation 7 as long as they contain the detail required by Schedule 4. Part 1 of Schedule 4 sets out the particulars to be kept in records of any event which is reportable under regulation 3 and these particulars are shown in *Box 14.2*. The particulars of reportable diseases which must be recorded under regulation 5 and which are set out in part 2 of Schedule 4 are shown in *Box 14.3*.

Box 14.2. Particulars to be kept in records of major injuries and death

- Date and time of the accident or dangerous occurrence
- Details of the person injured at work: full name; occupation; nature of injury
- Details of a person not at work: full name; status (e.g. customer, visitor); nature of injury
- Place where the accident or dangerous occurrence happened
- A brief description of the circumstances in which the accident or dangerous occurrence happened
- The date on which the event was first reported to the relevant enforcing authority
- The method by which the event was reported

Box 14.3. Particulars to be kept in records of diseases

- Date of diagnosis of the disease
- Name of the person affected
- Occupation of the person affected
- Name or nature of the disease
- The date on which the disease was first reported to the relevant enforcing authority
- The method by which the disease was reported

Source: HSE (2009)

Confidentiality and the accident book

The Information Commissioner in June 2003 allowed a seven-month lead-in time to ensure compliance of the Accident Book with Data Protection legislation. The HSE has published an Accident Book (B1510) which complies with Data Protection legislation. The new design allows for accidents to be recorded, while details of individuals can be stored separately in a secure location. Business premises had to comply with the new regulations by 31 December 2003.

Further information can be obtained from the Health and Safety Executive website devoted to RIDDOR (www.hse.gov.uk/riddor/index.htm).

Application of the law to *Scenario 14.1*

The major injury to Clematis is reportable under the RIDDOR regulations. The responsibility for the reporting lies upon the employer. The NHS trust should have ensured that there were in place procedures to ensure that reports were made in the approved way. Clematis may of course have been mistaken in assuming that there had been no notification of her injury, but it would be wise for her to make inquiries to discover who had reported the information.

Conclusions

There is still little evidence that the NHS is learning from the accidents to staff and patients and preventing a re-occurrence. However improvements in reporting mechanisms of all adverse events should ensure that the data are there to enable corrective action to be taken. The NHS Redress Act which is yet to be implemented did not contain a statutory duty of candour for staff to notify senior management and ultimately patients of all adverse events and in spite of the initiative of the National Patient Safety Agency to promote openness and honesty within the NHS there are still fears of considerable under-reporting of adverse incidents and hazards (*Chapter 13*). Lord Young's report has recommended changes to the time of absence from work after which an injury must be reported. As a consequence, the HSE opened a three month consultation on changes to RIDDOR on 31 January 2011. These, together with other changes proposed by Lord Young, are discussed in *Chapter 24*.

References

Health and Safety Executive (2000) *HSE wins funding for central incident reporting scheme. Press release E023:00* 16 February. HSE, Sheffield

Health and Safety Executive (2009) *Guide to the Reporting of Injuries, Disease and Dangerous Occurrence Regulations 1995* (3rd edn updated) HSE, Sheffield

Reporting of Injuries, Disease and Dangerous Occurrence Regulations 1995 SI 1995 No 3163 Stationery Office, London

CHAPTER 15

Infection control

Scenario 15.1. Dirty theatres

Sarah is an operating department practitioner working in the operating theatres. She is aware that the theatre is not being cleaned properly and therefore is concerned at the possibility of hospital-acquired infection. What action should she take?

Introduction

The level of infection and, in particular, hospital-acquired infections (HAIs), are of considerable concern. This chapter considers the reports on hospital acquired infection, the recommendations of the National Audit Office report, the Department of Health's NHS hospital clean-up campaign and the appointment of matrons. High standards of infection control are vital across the whole spectrum of health care. Ill people, babies and patients undergoing radiotherapy or chemotherapy and other treatments which depress the immune system are all extremely vulnerable to infections. Postoperative patients also need to receive protection from infections. Precautions must be taken to prevent the risk of cross-infection between patients and staff. In serious situations, this may require the closure of a department.

On the other hand, patients may themselves be suffering from infections and are liable to spread infections to other patients and to staff and any risk assessment needs to ensure that patients are checked on admission and all precautions taken to prevent the spread of infections brought into the hospital.

The highest standards of sterile practice and cleanliness are required and these can never be relaxed. Risk assessment and the management of cross-infections should be part of the basic philosophy of every department and ward with the person responsible for ensuring compliance clearly identified. This would be required by both statutory duties as well as the duties of the employer at common law and the occupier under the Occupier's Liability Act 1957 (see *Chapters 8 and 9*). Notifiable diseases are considered in the next chapter.

Meticillin-resistant *Staphylococcus aureus* (MRSA)

One of the greatest challenges for all those working in health care is the control and eradication of meticillin-resistant *Staphylococcus aureus* (MRSA). George Duckworth, of the Public Health Laboratory Service, stated that the proportion of all *S. aureus* bloodstream infections had increased from less than three percent before 1991 to 37 percent in 1999 (Leach 1999). This poses a major problem for all hospital and community health professionals. It appears to be accepted that it is not a problem which will ever be completely eradicated. Munro (1999) suggests that poor hygiene standards in hospitals are largely to blame for the increase in MRSA and other infections. The Royal College of Nursing has provided guidance for nurses on MRSA (Royal College of Nursing 2000). As well as identifying the features of MRSA, it considers the revised guidelines for control, the standard infection control precautions, additional precautions for MRSA, treatment of patients with MRSA, and community and communication issues. Mandatory reporting of MRSA began in April 2001. In recent years the number of reported deaths from MRSA have declined providing evidence of the improvements in cross-infection control in hospitals. Figures available from the National Statistics on-line were as follows:

The number of death certificates in England and Wales mentioning meticillin-resistant Staphylococcus aureus (MRSA) decreased by 37 percent in 2009 to 781 from 1230 in 2008. Deaths involving Staphylococcus aureus (including those which did not specify meticillin resistance) fell by 16 percent, from 1500 in 2008 to 1253 in 2009. On 19 percent of death certificates which mentioned MRSA in 2009, this infection was recorded as the underlying cause of death. This figure varied between 17 percent and 36 percent over the 1993–2009 period.

The Health Protection Agency estimated from survey data that about eight percent of patients in English hospitals had an HAI in 2006. A survey carried out by the National Opinion Poll (Hawkes 2002), showed that one in 10 patients leave hospital with an infection that they have picked up on the wards and that infections affect up to 710000 patients a year.

The Health Protection Agency (see below) published a Report in 2004 which pointed out that the number of people dying from the MRSA superbug had risen more than fifteen-fold in the past decade. It was directly responsible or an underlying cause of 800 deaths in 2002, compared with just 51 cases in 1993. Laboratory reports of MRSA blood poisoning also rose sharply over the same period from 210 cases to more than 5300. MRSA now affects more than 7000 hospital patients a year. MRSA Action UK has been set up to raise public awareness, campaign for safer standards and support sufferers and dependants. Its website is: mrsaactionuk.net.

National Audit Office report

A report by the National Audit Office (2000) has raised major concerns about the level of hospital-acquired infection (HAI). The report suggested that HAI could be the main or a contributory cause to 20000, or four percent, of deaths a year in the UK and that there are at least about 100000 cases of HAI with an estimated cost to the NHS of £1 billion. The National Audit Office drew conclusions on the strategic management of HAI, surveillance, the extent and cost of HAI, and the effectiveness of prevention, detection and control measures. Its recommendations include reviewing the factors listed in *Box 15.1*.

Box 15.1. Recommendations of the National Audit Office

- Consider the value of using an infection control manual
- Review the 1995 Guidance on Infection Control
- Consider the cost-effectiveness of screening patients and staff and isolation of patients together with standards and guidelines
- Review policies on provision of education and training
- Make arrangements for monitoring hospital hygiene and hospital practices
- Ensure advice on hand washing is implemented
- Review clinical audit arrangements to ensure infection control is covered
- Review isolation facilities
- Review guidance on management of HAI outbreaks

Government multipronged initiative to tackle hospital-acquired infections

Following the National Audit Office report the Government announced a multipronged initiative to tackle HAIs. Among the initiatives proposed were:

- An antimicrobial strategy including a clamp down on inappropriate antibiotic use and better infection control measures.

- Independent inspection of hospitals by the Audit Commission and Commission for Health Improvement (now the Care Quality Commission which replaced the Commission for Healthcare Audit and Inspection). The Government has stated that the Commission for Health Improvement and the Audit Commission would conduct ward inspections and be given the right to seek information on HAI and to publish it (Sherman 2000).
- The report on the NHS, commissioned by the Government, reported that it found grubby wards, litter-strewn entrances and dirty casualty departments throughout the NHS.

On 31 July 2000, Lord Hunt announced that NHS hospitals were to be given £150000 each to clean up their wards and disinfect bathrooms as part of a £31 million campaign. The money could be used for extra cleaning staff, materials, equipment and new towels and linen. Patient environment action teams would make unannounced inspections every six months and those hospitals which failed to meet standards would be 'named and shamed'. National standards for cleanliness would form part of performance assessment guidelines for hospitals. From July 2003, all NHS trusts have had to report any infections which are resistant to antibiotics, and any serious incidents arising from hospital infections. In addition in 2003 hospital pharmacists were given £12 million to monitor and control more carefully the use of antibiotics. The initiative will be monitored by the Specialist Advisory Committee on antimicrobial resistance (SACAR) (Department of Health 2003b).

Care Quality Commission (CQC)

The CQC replaced the Healthcare Commission, the Commission for Social Care Inspection and the Mental Health Act Commission in April 2009. On 13 April 2009 it made the following statement:

> Trusts are urged to remain vigilant and strive for further improvement. The Care Quality Commission today (Friday) commended the majority of NHS trusts for improving infection control. It pointed out that infection rates are falling and that many hospitals are continuing to strengthen systems for protecting patients. In the latest measure to drive improvement, it registered for the first time 388 NHS trusts to provide care after carrying out an assessment of whether they meet government regulations for managing infection. To carry out the assessment, it

asked that trusts declare whether they were compliant with the regulations and cross-checked this with other performance information, including patient and staff surveys, findings from the Healthcare Commission's hygiene inspections, trusts' declarations against core standards for infection control, and rates of MRSA and Clostridium difficile infection. While CQC registered all trusts, it made registration of 21 trusts subject to conditions, which are legally enforceable and must be met within agreed timescales or enforcement action will follow. It urged all 388 trusts to remain vigilant, ensure they complete planned programmes of improvement, and regularly review their performance.

In 2010 independent health care and adult social care was brought under the aegis of the CQC.

Evidence can be seen on the CQC website of the effectiveness of its strategy to improve standards of infection control. For example, on 13 July 2010 it published the following:

Mid Essex Services NHS Trust had made the necessary improvements to cleanliness and infection control and will now lift the condition it had imposed on the trust's registration. CQC imposed the condition on 1 April, when it introduced a tough new registration system for NHS trusts. Mid Essex was one of 22 trusts registered with conditions to improve aspects of quality and safety. The Commission had collected evidence from the hospital during an inspection on 12 February, which had shown that members of staff were not aware of policies to prevent and control infections and some areas were not adequately clean. It required the trust to take urgent action to ensure that its locations are clean and safe for patients, workers and others by operating an effective system to assess the risk, prevention, detection and control of the spread of healthcare associated infection. CQC set a deadline of 16 April for the trust to provide evidence that improvements were in place. To check whether the necessary improvements had been made, CQC made an unannounced site visit on 12 May, inspecting five wards as well as other areas of the trust. CQC found that cleanliness and infection control had improved. It reported that through observations of ward areas and staff interviews, no evidence was found that the trust has breached the regulation to protect patients, workers and others from the risks of acquiring a healthcare-associated infection. Staff were able to outline their responsibilities and processes to be followed for effective cleaning, prevention and management of potential needle and scalpel injuries. However CQC did see some areas for improvement, although the concerns were minor and did not amount to a

> breech:'with regard to the patient environment, there were areas that were dusty
> and were not as clean as they could have been, however these were minor.'
> There were some areas where the decontamination of moving and medical
> equipment, pillows and mattresses and disposable items needed to be better
> logged and records weren't as up to date as they could have been.

Clearly the power of the CQC to make unannounced visits, to set conditions with the underlying power to remove a health or social care organisation from its register is formidable in the battle to raise infection control standards.

Infectious diseases strategy

On 2nd January 2002, the Chief Medical Officer published a strategy for combating new diseases (Department of Health 2002b). The strategy identified HAI as a priority and new action plans were being developed (Department of Health 2002c). (The implementation plan relating to Hepatitis C is considered in *Chapter 16*.) One of the most significant recommendations was that a new Health Protection Agency (HPA) (see below) was to be established to streamline the services involved in the prevention and control of infectious diseases. It was set up in the light of the report of the Chief Medical Officer of Health, *Getting Ahead of the Curve* (2002), which recognised the need to bring together in one organisation the skills and expertise in a number of organisations to work in a more co-ordinated way, to reduce the burden and consequences of health protection threats or disease with the aim of providing a more comprehensive and effective response to threats to the public's health. The agency was to provide an integrated approach to all aspects of health protection and would combine the functions of the following national bodies:

- Public Health Laboratory Service (including the Communicable Disease Surveillance Centre and Central Public Health Laboratory).
- National Radiological Protection Board.
- Centre for Applied Microbiology and Research.
- National Focus for Chemical Incidents.
- The Regional Service Provider Units that support the management of chemical incidents.
- The National Poisons Information Service.
- NHS public health staff responsible for infectious disease control, emergency planning, and other protection support.

Other proposals are shown in *Box 15.2*.

The strategy also reviews why the prevalence and control of infectious disease can be unpredictable and difficult to manage and sets out a number of key priorities for action. These include intensifying control measures against tuberculosis and other diseases and identifying more links between infectious and chronic diseases. A long-term strategy to prevent and reduce health care-associated infections (HCAIs) was published by the Chief Medical Officer in September 2003.

Box 15.2. Strategy for infectious diseases: Proposals

- National expert panel to assess the threat from new and emerging infectious diseases
- Strengthened and expanded system of infectious disease surveillance
- Programme of new vaccine development
- A new inspector of microbiology
- A set of action plans to intensify control measures for specific diseases

---

Strategy *Winning Ways*

In December 2003, the Chief Medical Officer published a report, *Winning Ways,* which is available on the Department of Health website (http://www.dh.gov.uk/ PublicationsAndStatistics). At the same time a table of MRSA rate per 1000 bed days was published. This showed rates varying from York Health Services at 0.04 to Weston Area Health at 0.30. In specialist hospitals the rate varied from Liverpool Women's Hospital at 0.05 to the University Hospital Birmingham at 0.49. In single specialist hospitals the range was from Moorfields Eye Hospital with 0.00 to Papworth Hospital 0.45 (Lister 2003). *Winning Ways* set out a strategy to reduce infections in health care. The plans included:

- Creating a directory of infection control in every NHS trust to impose tough new rules.
- A dedicated infection control team in each NHS trust.
- A new system which has cut food poisoning in the catering trade is to be introduced in the NHS.
- A new drive to ensure staff follow basic techniques for cutting infection

rates through frequent handwashing and disinfection.

- Reducing the use of catheters and drips (procedures most likely to cause infection).
- Commission for Health Audit and Inspection (CHAI) (now CQC) to make infection control a key priority when compiling its star ratings of trusts.
- £3 million would be spent on research and development on hospital-acquired infections.
- Increasing the number of single rooms in new hospitals, so that new patients could be screened for MRSA or those with MRSA could be isolated.

Matrons

Modern matrons were introduced into the NHS by the Department of Health in 2001. A progress report by the Department of Health (2002d) stated that nearly 2000 matrons had been appointed. The aim was that every hospital should have a matron in overall charge of a group of wards. They would be responsible for:

- Driving up standards of care.
- Ensuring wards are clean.
- Ensuring patients are fed properly.
- Helping to set and monitor standards for cleaning and catering.
- Having authority to take action where these are not met.

It was intended that matrons should be strong clinical leaders with distinctive uniforms to ensure that they are visible to patients and their families.

In Appendix 1 to the Department of Health report (2004b) (see below) on progress so far, it is stated that over 3000 matrons have been appointed since 1999 and over £14 million had been invested in ward housekeepers. There have been concerns as to how effective the modern matrons have been. An article in the *Journal of Infection Prevention* by Koteyko and Nerlich (2008) identifies problems that challenge this model of the modern matron and links them to possible problems in infection control.

The study describes cases of difficulty in fulfilling leadership requirements because of organisational barriers to empowerment despite arguments to the contrary. Unless a significant budgetary responsibility is made, part of the modern matron's role, personal skills (communication, problem solving) alone may not be sufficient to sustain it and may not lead to achieving control over infection, which was the initial trigger for instituting this role.

An article in the *Nursing Times* also questioned whether they had made a difference (Mooney 2008).

Standard principles for preventing hospital-acquired infections

The Department of Health has published standard principles for preventing HAIs (Pratt et al 2001). The principles provide guidance on infection control precautions that should be applied by all health care practitioners to the care of all hospital inpatients all the time. The recommendations cover four distinct interventions:

* Hospital environment hygiene.
* Hand hygiene.
* The use of personal protective equipment.
* The use and disposal of sharps.

Each intervention is supported by relevant research evidence of its efficacy.

National standards of cleanliness for the NHS

In 2002, the NHS Estates within the Department of Health published a guide for national standards of cleanliness for the NHS (NHS Estates 2002). This publication enables hospital staff to monitor and improve the cleaning services. In a commentary on the national standards for cleanliness, Castledine (2002) notes the emphasis on the nurse's role in ensuring that things get done and that audit is carried out and that hospitals improve their cleanliness, and welcomes the return to one of the most important aspects of hospital nursing care.

Testing of staff

The battle to reduce HAIs and control the level of cross-infection in hospitals is likely to remain at the forefront of Department of Health strategic planning. As part of this strategy, the Department of Health announced, on 2 January 2003, draft guidance for carrying out health checks for new health care staff for serious communicable diseases in order to provide greater protection for patients (Department of Health 2003a). Those new staff whose jobs involve exposure-prone procedures (EPPs) (e.g. surgery, obstetrics and gynaecology, dentistry and midwifery) will have to test negative for human immunodeficiency virus (HIV) and hepatitis B and C before taking up such a post. Other new staff whose work does not involve EPPs will also be offered testing for hepatitis C and HIV. All new staff are already tested for hepatitis B and tuberculosis screening. (For further details on protection of staff and patients from HIV see *Chapter 16*.)

Developments in tackling MRSA

New MRSA figures were published in July 2004 by the Department of Health and Health Protection Agency (Department of Health 2004a) which showed that reports of MRSA infections had increased by 3.6 percent in the last year, being the third year in which mandatory surveillance for monitoring MRSA had been in place. At the same time a report from the National Audit Office (2004) was published in which the NAO concluded that the implementation of its recommendations published in 2000 had been patchy. The NAO accepted that the priority given to infection control had increased but concluded that despite some local improvements in information, the NHS still lacked sufficient information on the extent and cost of hospital acquired infection and further action was required using a range of approaches to change staff behaviour to reduce its risks. The NAO considered that the increased throughput of patients to meet performance targets had resulted in considerable pressure towards higher bed occupancy which is not always consistent with good infection control and bed management practices.

In the light of this information, the Secretary of State for Health announced new initiatives to tackle MRSA and hospital-acquired infection (Department of Health 2004b). *Towards Cleaner Hospitals and Lower Rates of Infection* envisaged a campaign for action based on the following principles:

- Being open with the public.
- Giving power to patients.
- A matron's charter.
- Independent inspection to measure progress.
- Learning from the very best.
- Harnessing the latest research and technology.

The campaign envisaged that Patient Forums would be invited to undertake cleanliness inspections and report their findings to the public four times a year. The NPSA (see *Chapter 13*) announced in 2004 that it had appointed a permanent infection control specialist to its safety solutions directorate. Julie Storr from the Oxford Radcliffe hospitals was seconded to the NPSA for a year to lead the Clean Your Hands campaign (www.npsa.nhs.uk).

Code of practice

The Government published the first code of practice for the NHS regarding HCAIs in 2006. All NHS trusts that provide regulated activities must be registered with the Care Quality Commission (see above) and to do so they must meet a range of Government regulations, including one on cleanliness and infection control. To meet legal requirements, NHS trusts must ensure that patients, workers and others are protected against the identifiable risks of acquiring an HCAI. To help NHS trusts to ensure they follow good practices for infection control and meet the regulation, the Department of Health published an updated version of the code of practice regarding HCAIs on 1 April 2010, under the Health and Social Care Act 2008. This is called the *Code of Practice for Health and Adult Social Care on the Prevention and Control of Infections and Related Guidance*. The code of practice lists 10 criteria that are used to judge whether an NHS trust is compliant with the regulation regarding cleanliness and infection control.

The CQC on its website describes the code of practice as follows:

These criteria are designed to ensure that patients are cared for in a clean environment, where the risks of HCAIs are kept as low as possible. They cover all aspects of infection control, not only cleanliness.

Examples of good practices in the code of practice are:

- Having staff members who are dedicated to overseeing infection control.
- Providing the right kind of hand-washing facilities in the right places, and antibacterial hand rub.
- Having arrangements for the thorough cleaning (decontamination) of instruments and other equipment.
- Having enough isolation facilities, so the risk of infections spreading between patients is minimised.
- Ensuring the prudent use of antimicrobial drugs, as some can increase the risk of patients acquiring an HCAI.

The CQC states that it has now integrated the monitoring of trusts' compliance with the essential standard on cleanliness and infection control into its overall approach for monitoring compliance with all essential standards of safety and quality.

Health Protection Agency (HPA)

Under the Health Protection Agency Act 2004 a corporate body known as the Health Protection Agency has been set up with the following functions:

- The protection of the community (or any part of the community) against infectious disease and other dangers to health.
- The prevention of the spread of infectious disease.
- The provision of assistance to any other person who exercises functions in relation to the matters mentioned in the above paragraphs.
- Other such functions in relation to health as the Secretary of State or the Welsh Assembly directs (after consultation with each other).

Supplementary functions include:

- Engaging in or commissioning research.
- Obtaining and analysing data and other information.
- Providing laboratory services.
- Providing other technical and clinical services.
- Providing training in relation to matters in respect of which the agency has functions.
- Making available to any other body such persons, materials and facilities as it thinks appropriate.
- Providing information and advice.

Schedule 1 sets out the membership of the Agency and their terms of and procedures for appointment, rules relating to proceedings, staff and finance. An annual report must be prepared and sent to the Secretary of State.

Further information on the work of the HPA together with copies of its news letters and minutes of its meetings is available on the website (www.dh.gov.uk/cmo/hpa/index.htm).

The HPA prides itself on its independence:

People want clear, unambiguous and authoritative information on public health protection issues from an independent source, which they feel they can trust. The Health Protection Agency will give impartial advice to the public, professionals and government alike, which is based on the experience and expertise of the professionals working in the organisation.

Radiation protection functions

The HPA also has functions in relation to risks connected with radiation including the advancement of the acquisition of knowledge about protection from such risks and the provision of information and advice in relation to the protection of the community or any part of the community. It took over the functions of the National Radiological Protection Board.

Co-operation with other bodies

Under section 5 the HPA has a statutory duty to cooperate with other bodies which exercise functions relating to health or any other matter in relation to which the Agency also exercises functions.

Standards

The HPA is treated as a NHS body for the purpose of being subject to standards set by the Secretary of State under the Health and Social Care (Community Health and Standards) Act 2003.

Emergency response

The plans of the HPA to meet a possible terrorist emergency or potential SARS outbreak or other emergency include the following:

- Build on the existing major incident plans.
- Develop the infrastructure for surveillance and early recognition of events.
- Continue to produce guidance for health protection for these new hazards.
- Identify specific countermeasures, making sure that they are available quickly.
- Provide training and test new plans.
- Co-ordinate the Health Protection Agency's divisions and expertise in emergency situations.

The hope was that the different divisions within the HPA would co-operate together to enable integration at local, regional and national levels which was not so easy when they were separate organisations. The HPA was to be the single identifiable health protection organisation for the NHS, Government and other agencies.

Future of the HPA

In the review of Arms' Length Bodies carried out by the Coalition Government in 2010 (Department of Health 2010) it is proposed that the Health Protection Agency and the National Treatment Centre will be abolished as statutory organisations and their functions will be transferred to the Secretary of State as part of the new Public Health Service. The new Public Health Service will be directly accountable to the Secretary of State, and will integrate and streamline existing health improvement and protection bodies and functions, with an increased emphasis on research, analysis and evaluation. At the time of writing the new Public Health Service is still to be established.

SARS

The UK was fortunate, compared with the Far East and Canada, in not having to face an outbreak of the SARS infection. However, the Department of Health was concerned at the ability of this country to deal with such an outbreak and introduced legislation for new powers to be given to doctors to control the spread of that or a similar disease. Provisions were accordingly made in the Health and Social Care Act 2008.

Health and Social Care Act 2008

Part 3 of the Health and Social Care Act 2008 made significant changes to the laws relating to Public Health including giving to the Secretary of State powers to make regulations governing international travel and also to prevent or control the spread of contamination or infection in England and Wales. A new Part 2A of the Public Health (Control of Diseases) Act 1984 replaces the existing Part 2. Other changes to the Public Health (Control of Disease) Act 1984 are considered in *Chapter 16*.

Application of the law to *Scenario 15.1*

Sarah has every right to be concerned. Patients following surgery are vulnerable to infections and it is essential that Sarah takes action to ensure that the situation is remedied. She should attempt to obtain a copy of the NHS Estates publication on national standards of cleanliness for the NHS and the tools suggested in that publication could assist her in formulating her concerns. Her next step should be to raise her concerns with the operating theatres manager. The manager may refer her, if such a person exists, to a matron, who would have a responsibility to raise the issue of cleanliness standards with senior management, involving the control of an infection officer. Alternatively if there is a Director of Infection Control in the hospital, that person could be informed. It may be that cleaning services are undertaken by an outside firm and there is inadequate supervision and enforcement of contractual standards. If Sarah finds that no-one appears to be interested sufficiently to take on board her concerns and ensure action is taken, then she should put her concerns in writing and make use of the whistle-blowing procedure which her trust should have in place. If she follows the procedure in making her concerns known she is protected against any victimisation. Whistle-blowing is considered in *Chapter 23*.

Conclusions

There are signs that progress is being made in the fight to control hospital-acquired infection. Rates of MRSA infection have declined and the clean hands campaign appears to be working. However continued vigilance is constantly required. The Care Quality Commission, with stronger enforcement powers than its predecessors, has considerable responsibility in ensuring that standards of cross-infection control are maintained across the NHS and can take appropriate action when there are signs of failure.

References

Castledine G (2002) Hospitals are to be given standards of cleanliness. *British Journal of Nursing* **11**(8): 590

Chief Medical Officer of Health (2002) *Getting Ahead of the Curve*. Department of Health, London

Chief Medical Officer of Health (2003) *Winning Ways: Working together to reduce health-care associated infection in England*. DoH, London

Department of Health (2002a) *Lord Hunt Welcomes Report into Rates of MRSA Hospital Infection by NHS Trust*. Press release 0066. DoH, London

Department of Health (2002b) *Getting Ahead of the Curve: A Strategy for Combating Infectious Diseases (including other aspects of health promotion)*. DoH, London

Department of Health (2002c) *Chief Medical Officer Launches Infectious Disease Strategy*. Press release 0013. DoH, London

Department of Health (2002d) *Modern Matrons in the NHS — A Progress Report*. DoH,

London

Department of Health (2003a) *Health Clearance for Serious Communicable Diseases: New Health Care Workers*. DoH, London (www.dh.gov.uk/healthclear)

Department of Health (2003b) *CMO to step up fight against hospital infections*. Press Release 9 June 2003

Department of Health (2004a) *New MRSA figures published 2004/0261*, DoH, London

Department of Health (2004b) *Towards cleaner hospital and lower rates of infection. A summary of action*. DoH, London

Department of Health (2010) *Liberating the NHS: Report of the Arm's Length Bodies*. DoH, London

Hawkes N (2002) Hospitals dirtier than abattoirs says report. *The Times* 16 May

Health Protection Agency (2004) *Report on MRSA*. HPA, London

Koteyko N, Nerlich B (2008) Modern matrons and infection control practices: Aspirations and realities. *Journal of Infection Prevention* **9**(2): 18–22

Leach E (1999) Resistance fighters. *Nursing Times* **95**(38): 18

Lister S (2003) Worst trust defends record. *The Times*, 6 December

Mooney H (2008) Are Modern Matrons making a difference? *Nursing Times* **104**(24): 8–9

Munro R (1999) Clean up your act. *Nursing Times* **96**(25): 26–7

National Audit Office (2000) *The management and control of hospital-acquired infection in acute NHS Trusts in England*. The Stationery Office, London

National Audit Office (2004) *Improving patient care by reducing the risk of hospital acquired infection: A progress report. HC 876 Session 2003–4*. The Stationery Office, London

NHS Estates (2002) *National Standards of Cleanliness for the NHS*. The Stationery Office, London

Pratt RJ, Pellow C, Loveday HP et al (2001) The epic project: Developing national evidence-based guidelines for preventing healthcare associated infections. Phase I: Guidelines for preventing hospital-acquired infections. *Journal of Hospital Infection* **47**(supplement): S21–37

Public Health (Infectious Diseases) Regulations 1988 (SI 1988 No 1546)

Public Health Laboratory Service (2002) *Communicable Disease Report*. Public Health Laboratory Service, London

Royal College of Nursing (2000) *Methicillin-resistant Staphylococcus Aureus*. Royal College of Nursing, London

Sherman J (2000) Infections caught in hospital to be exposed. *The Times* 13 June

CHAPTER 16

Laws relating to notifiable diseases and HIV/AIDS

Scenario 16.1. Keeping positive HIV a secret

Following a holiday in Africa, Brenda, an orthoptist, was told that she had probably been infected with the human immunodeficiency virus. She felt reasonably fit and since she worked in ophthalmic outpatients, an area where there was a very low risk of infecting patients, she wanted to keep this information to herself. What is the law?

Introduction

In the last chapter the problems relating to cross-infection and the law relating to liability were considered. In this chapter the statutory provisions relating to notifiable diseases are considered together with the guidance and laws relating to human immunodeficiency virus/acquired immunodeficiency syndrome (HIV/AIDS). The legal rights of the employee in relation to HIV/AIDS are also considered.

Notification of infectious diseases

Diseases that are notifiable are shown in *Boxes 16.1 and 16.2*. Schedule 1 covers those notifiable diseases that come under the duties set by the Public Health (Control of Disease) Act 1984 and are set out in Schedule 1 of the Health Protection (Notification) Regulations 2010. These diseases must be reported to the local authority. Those diseases under Schedule 2 are covered by Regulation 4 of the Health Protection (Notification) Regulations 2010 (SI 2010/659) and the 1984 Act applies to a more limited extent. (Regulation 4 relates to the duty on diagnostic laboratories to report causative agents found in human samples.)

Procedure for notification

Under section 11 of the 1984 Act, registered medical practitioners have a duty to notify the proper office of the local authority if they become aware, or suspect,

---

Box 16.1. Notifiable diseases: Schedule I

Acute encephalitis
Acute infectious hepatitis
Acute meningitis
Acute poliomyelitis
Anthrax
Botulism
Brucellosis
Cholera
Diphtheria
Enteric fever (typhoid or
  paratyphoid fever)
Food poisoning
Haemolytic uraemic

syndrome (HUS)
Infectious bloody
  diarrhoea
Invasive group A
  streptococcal disease
  and scarlet fever
Legionnaires' disease
Leprosy
Malaria
Measles
Meningococcal
  septicaemia
Mumps

Plague
Rabies
Rubella
SARS
Smallpox
Tetanus
Tuberculosis
Typhus
Viral haemorrhagic fever
  (VHF)
Whooping cough
Yellow fever

---

that a patient whom they are attending within the district of a local authority is suffering from a notifiable disease or from food poisoning. The duty does not apply if they believe, and have reasonable grounds for believing, that some other registered medical practitioner has complied with the duty.

- Under the 2010 Regulation 2(1) A registered medical practitioner (R) must notify the proper officer of the relevant local authority where R has reasonable grounds for suspecting that a patient (P) whom R is attending
  (a) Has a notifiable disease;
  (b) Has an infection which, in the view of R, presents or could present significant harm to human health; or
  (c) Is contaminated in a manner which, in the view of R, presents or could present significant harm to human health.

Information that must be passed on is as follows:

- Regulation 2(2): The notification must include the following information insofar as it is known to R
  (a) P's name, date of birth and sex;
  (b) P's home address including postcode;

Box 16.2. Notifiable diseases: Schedule 2

Bacillus anthracis
Bacillus cereus (only if associated with food poisoning)
Bordetella pertussis
Borrelia spp
Brucella spp
Burkholderia mallei
Burkholderia pseudomallei
Campylobacter spp
Chikungunya virus
Chlamydophila psittaci
Clostridium botulinum
Clostridium perfringens (only if associated with food poisoning)
Clostridium tetani
Corynebacterium diphtheriae
Corynebacterium ulcerans
Coxiella burnetii
Crimean-Congo haemorrhagic fever virus
Cryptosporidium spp
Dengue virus
Ebola virus
Entamoeba histolytica

Francisella tularensis
Giardia lamblia
Guanarito virus
Haemophilus influenzae (invasive)
Hanta virus
Hepatitis A, B, C, delta, and E viruses
Influenza virus
Junin virus
Kyasanur Forest disease virus
Lassa virus
Legionella spp
Leptospira interrogans
Listeria monocytogenes
Machupo virus
Marburg virus
Measles virus
Mumps virus
Mycobacterium tuberculosis complex
Neisseria meningitidis
Omsk haemorrhagic fever virus
Plasmodium falciparum, vivax, ovale, malariae, knowlesi

Polio virus (wild or vaccine types)
Rabies virus (classical rabies and rabies-related lyssaviruses)
Rickettsia spp
Rift Valley fever virus
Rubella virus
Sabia virus
Salmonella spp
SARS coronavirus
Shigella spp
Streptococcus pneumoniae (invasive)
Streptococcus pyogenes (invasive)
Varicella zoster virus
Variola virus
Verocytotoxigenic Escherichia coli (including E.coli O157)
Vibrio cholerae
West Nile Virus
Yellow fever virus
Yersinia pestis

(c) P's current residence (if not home address);
(d) P's telephone number;
(e) P's NHS number;
(f) P's occupation (if R considers it relevant);
(g) The name, address and postcode of P's place of work or education (if R considers it relevant);

    (h) P's relevant overseas travel history;

    (i)   P's ethnicity;

    (j)   Contact details for a parent of P (where P is a child);

    (k) The disease or infection which P has or is suspected of having or the nature of P's contamination or suspected contamination;

    (l)   The date of onset of P's symptoms;

    (m) The date of R's diagnosis; and

    (n) R's name, address and telephone number.

- **Regulation 2(3)** The notification must be provided in writing within 3 days beginning with the day on which R forms a suspicion under Regulation 2(1).

- **Regulation 2(4)** Without prejudice to Regulation 2(3), if R considers that the case is urgent, notification must be provided orally as soon as reasonably practicable.

- **Regulation 2(5)** In determining whether the case is urgent, R must have regard to

      (a) The nature of the suspected disease, infection or contamination;

      (b) The ease of spread of that disease, infection or contamination;

      (c)   The ways in which the spread of the disease, infection or contamination can be prevented or controlled; and

      (d) P's circumstances (including age, sex and occupation).

          Public Health (Control of Disease) Act 1984 Section 11 as amended by The Health Protection (Notification) Regulations 2010 No. 659

N.B. Section 11(4) imposes a criminal sanction on a person who fails to comply with an obligation imposed on him under the provisions set out above)

As noted in *Chapter 15* and above, the Health and Social Care Act 2008 made significant changes to the Public Health Act 1984 and subsequent regulations. A new Part 2A replaces Part 2 of the 1984 Act in accordance with Section 129 of the 2008 Act. Part 2A covers the following sections:

- Section 129 replaces part 2 of the 1984 Act with Part 2A as follows:

45A   Infection or contamination

45B   Health protection regulations: International travel etc.

45C   Health protection regulations: Domestic

45D Restrictions on power to make regulations under section 45C
45E Medical treatment
45F Health protection regulations: Supplementary
45G Power to order health measures in relation to persons
45H Power to order health measures in relation to things
45I Power to order health measures in relation to premises
45J Orders in respect of groups
45K Part 2A orders: Supplementary
45L Period for which Part 2A order may be in force
45M Procedure for making, varying and revoking Part 2A orders
45N Power to make further provision by regulations
45O Enforcement of Part 2A orders
45P General provision about regulations
45Q Parliamentary control
45R Emergency procedure
45S Application to territorial sea
45T Part 2A: Further definitions

• Section 130: Further amendments relating to public health protection

(1) Part 2 of the Public Health (Control of Disease) Act 1984 (c. 22) (which is superseded by the new Part 2A inserted by section 129) ceases to have effect.

(2) Schedule 11 (which contains further amendments of that Act and other Acts) has effect.

The Act can be accessed on the Office of Public Information website.

Prevalence of AIDS/HIV

Figures issued by the Public Health Laboratory Service in November 2002 (Browne 2002), show a rapid growth in the number of new cases of persons identified as HIV positive. There were 2945 new cases in the first nine months of 2002, compared with 2354 in the previous year. This rise was considered to be mainly explained by the growth in HIV-positive people immigrating to the UK. Since there has been a drive to recruit workers from overseas to fill nursing and other vacancies in the NHS, there have been calls that there should be compulsory HIV testing for new NHS employees from overseas. As a consequence of the unlinked anonymous prevalence monitoring programme, an annual report on the prevalence of HIV and hepatitis infections is published each year by the Department of Health and is available from its website (www.dh.gov.uk/hivhepatitis/report). Figures provided by the Health Protection Agency in November 2003 showed that the number of people infected with HIV in Britain was increasing by nearly 20 percent a year, and one third were unaware that they have the disease. Fifty thousand people in Britain were HIV positive, up from 41 700 in 2002. In February 2004, the Health Protection Agency said that the number of new cases of HIV had risen by 20 percent in one year and most of the infections were contracted abroad (HPA website). Worldwide the annual death from AIDS has reached three million (Henderson 2003). The World Health Organization (WHO) estimated that 40 million people around the world were living with HIV or AIDS, including 2.5 million children below the age of 17 years. In December 2003, the WHO stated that the role of infected needles in spreading HIV had been underestimated: unsafe injections may be responsible for between a third and half of all cases in Africa, and not the 2.5 percent official figure (*The Times* 2004).

In 2011 the HPA reported on the largest ever annual number of new HIV diagnoses in men having sex with men (MSM) in the United Kingdom. It stated on its website that:

> Recently published data show that in 2010, an estimated 6750 people (4590 men and 2160 women) were first diagnosed with HIV in the United Kingdom, after adjusting the observed number of 6136 diagnoses for reporting delay. This represents a rate of 15.7 new diagnoses per 100000 population aged from 15 to 59 years (21.4 per 100000 men and 10.1 per 100000 women). The 2010 total was a slight increase on the number of new diagnoses seen in 2009, following a four year decline from the peak of 7837 diagnoses reported in 2005. Half of all those diagnosed in 2010 (50 percent; 3350) probably acquired their infection through heterosexual contact and 46 percent (3080) through sex between men (MSM).

It was estimated in 2009 that more than a quarter of those infected were unaware of the infection. In the light of the number of people unaware that they had the infection, the Regional Director for the Health Protection Agency in Yorkshire and the Humber, said:

> Whilst the figures indicate that rates of HIV are lower in our region when compared to most other areas of the UK, we're very concerned that a large number of people in our region remain unaware of their HIV status and that

national figures show half of all newly diagnosed people are being diagnosed late. We would like to see more people in our region being tested for HIV. This is crucial to reduce the number of people who are unaware of their HIV status and to increase the chances of early diagnosis, when treatment has a better chance of being successful.

In 2011 the National Institute for Health and Clinical Excellence (NICE 2011a) published guidance on increasing the uptake of HIV testing among black Africans in England and also guidance on increasing the uptake of testing of men who have sex with men (NICE 2011b). Both publications can be found on the NICE website (www.nice.org.uk/guidance).

The Health Protection Agency also publishes the Survey of Prevalent HIV Infections Diagnosed (SOPHID). This survey began in 1995 and is a cross-sectional survey of all individuals with diagnosed HIV infection who attend for HIV-related care within the NHS in England, Wales, and Northern Ireland within a calendar year. SOPHID is funded by the Department of Health and the London Specialised Commissioning Group (LSCG) and is conducted by the Heath Protection Agency's Centre for Infections. Scottish data are collected separately in Scotland by Health Protection Scotland (formerly SCIEH), and is incorporated into UK totals. The survey is run twice a year in London and annually outside London. Further information on SOPHID including answers to frequently asked questions is available on the HPA website. On 7 April 2011 (World Health Day) the World Health Organization (2011) issued a fact sheet on HIV drug resistance which highlighted the need for further surveillance and monitoring.

Statutory provisions for HIV/AIDS

HIV/AIDS infections come under the AIDS (Control) Act 1987, which requires periodical reports to be delivered to the regional health authority and the Secretary of State, containing the information listed in *Box 16.3*. The AIDS (Control) (Contents of Reports) Order 1988 extended this information to include that relating to HIV-positive persons. This information is required to enable the appropriate resources to be allocated and plans to be made. Under the Public Health (Infectious Diseases) Regulations 1988, local authorities have the power to apply to a Justice of the Peace (JP) for the removal of an AIDS sufferer to hospital to be detained there. The JP is also given the power to make an order for a person believed to be suffering from AIDS to be medically examined. There are also powers in relation to the disposal of the body of an AIDS sufferer.

Box 16.3. Information to be provided under the AIDs (Control) Act 1987

- The number of persons known to be persons with AIDS and the timing of the diagnosis
- The particulars of facilities and services to cope with HIV/AIDS provided by each authority
- The numbers of persons employed by the authority in providing such facilities
- Future provision over the next 12 months
- Action taken to educate members of the public in relation to AIDS and HIV, to provide training for testing for HIV/AIDS, and for the treatment, counselling and care of persons with AIDS or infected with HIV

The HIV/AIDS patient

The health professional is unable to refuse to care for a patient who is suffering from AIDS or who is HIV-positive. A survey of attitudes of practitioners to HIV/AIDS patients reported that 37 percent specifically argued that nurses should be allowed to refuse to care for a patient who had developed AIDS (Akinsanya and Rouse 1992). Professional practice and also the legal duty would, however, not permit a health professional to refuse. He/she could be dismissed from a job, removed from the professional register and possibly sued by a patient who suffered harm. Also, a health professional cannot insist that a patient suspected of being an HIV/AIDS carrier is compulsorily tested. This is not necessarily a disadvantage to the health professional, since it is possible to have false negatives, and if the patient has only recently picked up the infection it may not be shown up on testing, yet the patient could still transmit the disease.

The safest practice is to assume that every patient is a potential carrier and systems of work should be based on that risk.

Duty of care to the employee

An employee is entitled to all reasonable care being taken for his/her safety against reasonably foreseeable risks and dangers. The danger of contracting HIV/AIDS infection is one which could be regarded as reasonably foreseeable. This means the employer must take all reasonable care in terms of ensuring that a safe system of work is followed, that staff are trained and competent, and that equipment, facilities, buildings and the working environment are safe. The employer's duty derives both from the contract of employment and also from the criminal law and the laws relating to health and safety at work. These duties are enforced through the criminal courts (by prosecution under health and safety legislation) and the civil courts (by actions by employees for compensation for breach of contract) (see *Chapters 5 and 6*).

As it is unknown which patients are likely to be a danger to the health professional, it is important that every patient is treated as a potential source of infection and that the same high standards are followed for every case.

Duty to the HIV/AIDS client

If health professionals know that one of their clients is suffering from AIDS or is HIV-positive, what action should they take? Hopefully, their standards of care and safety are such that they would not have to take any additional precautions. The fact that the patient is an HIV carrier or sufferer from AIDS in no way reduces the duty of care that the health professional owes him/her. Indeed, in some ways it is higher because of the additional information that the health professional should be giving the patient about AIDS/HIV treatment and services.

Rights of HIV mothers

The case in *Box 16.4* came to light when a GP carrying out a routine check-up read in the mother's notes that she was HIV-positive and raised the issue with Camden Borough Council, bringing her case under the Children Act 1989. In cases involving children, 'the welfare of the child is the paramount consideration', and is the fundamental principle. In applying this principle to the facts, the judge ordered the baby to be tested for the HIV virus despite the opposition of her parents. While the judge ruled that an HIV test could be carried out, he did not rule that the mother should stop breast-feeding the child, even though breast-feeding the baby by an HIV mother is considered to double the chance of the baby contracting the disease (*Re C (HIV test)* [1999]).

Routine testing for HIV

Government policy announced on 13 August 1999 by the then Minister of Health, Tessa Jowell, for all pregnant women to be encouraged to have a routine HIV

Box 16.4. An HIV-positive mother

An HIV-positive mother refused to allow her four-month-old baby to be tested for the HIV virus. Both parents believed that HIV does not cause AIDS and that the conventional medical treatment of the virus did more harm than good. Judge Wilson noted that both parents were devoted to the baby and that they were knowledgeable and concerned about HIV. However, the judge accepted the current medical view that HIV could lead to AIDS and that drug therapy could be given to minimise the effect of the virus. The mother had refused to accept medical advice to have her baby delivered via a Caesarean section and to not breast-feed the baby. Instead, she arranged for a home delivery and was breast-feeding the baby.

---

test, is likely to increase the numbers of babies found to be infected and therefore the potential for parental disputes over babies being tested (Baldwin and Murray 1999). Two and a half percent of the newly reported HIV cases in 2000 were mother-to-baby infections (Baldwin and Murray 1999). The laws of consent still apply and a pregnant woman could refuse to be tested and, if she agrees, should be counselled before the testing.

The laws of consent to testing also apply to potential employees. An applicant for a post could not be compelled to undergo HIV/AIDS testing, although an offer of a job contract could be subject to a condition that the employee undergoes a medical examination.

The HIV/AIDS health professional

A health professional who becomes aware that he or she is HIV/AIDS infected has a duty to inform his or her employer. The former UKCC (now replaced by the Nursing and Midwifery Council) issued guidance for practitioners in relation to HIV/AIDS (UKCC 1992). A position article on HIV/AIDS was published by the Royal College of Midwives (Royal College of Midwives 1998). The Department of Health issued guidance on HIV/AIDS-infected healthcare workers (Department of Health 1999 updated 2005). In the past, the policy has been that patients will be told if they have been cared for by a person with HIV (UKCC 1992). This policy has now been changed and it was announced in November 2002 (Department of Health 2002) that in future there will no longer be a blanket policy that all patients cared for by a health worker found to be HIV-positive will be notified of this fact. Instead, the need to inform patients of any HIV transmission risk will be assessed on a case-by-case basis. The reason for this change of policy is that HIV transmission from a health care worker to a patient had never been recorded in the UK. Therefore, the risk of such infection is so low that the Department of Health considered that the notification policy should be reviewed. Telling patients of such a slim risk is seen as causing unnecessary anxiety. The Department of Health discussed with health professionals the revised guidelines, including defining which clinical procedures pose a transmission risk, and they were published in 2003 (Department of Health 2003a).

Because of the fact that such a high proportion of HIV/AIDS infections are contracted abroad, the Department of Health published a consultation document on health clearance for serious communicable diseases in 2003 (Department of Health 2003b).

Midwives

The midwife is one of the few health professionals subject to a statutory duty to agree to a medical examination (Nursing and Midwifery Council 2002). This means that if the midwife is suspected of being HIV/AIDS-infected then her employers or supervisor could legitimately request the local supervising authority to arrange for a test to be taken. There is not a similar statutory duty placed on other health professionals. However, all registered health professionals would have a professional duty to notify their registration body and also their employers that they were suffering from AIDS or were HIV-positive.

Rights of the HIV/AIDs health professional not to be identified

While health professionals would have a duty to notify the employer of the fact that they were HIV/AIDS-positive, the policy has been to protect the anonymity of health service employees and the courts have supported the confidentiality of employees' identity. A case in 1988 protected the confidentiality of the names of the health professionals who were found to be HIV-positive against public disclosure (*X v. Y and others* [1988]). The Court of Appeal advised that an injunction against disclosure of the health worker's identity should not be drawn up in too wide terms (*X v. Y and others* [1988]). In a case where a health professional appealed against a judge's order that the worker's health authority could be identified and that an earlier order restraining a newspaper from soliciting information should be set aside, the Court of Appeal held that while the health authority could not be identified, the health professional's specialty could be made known. The terms of the original order had been a Draconian fetter on the freedom of expression; the terms of the order had been too wide to be justified and it was not appropriate to reinstate it (*H (A healthcare worker) v. Associated Newspapers Ltd; H (A healthcare worker) v. N (A health authority)* [2002]).

Application of the law to *Scenario 16.1*

Brenda should be aware that she should notify her employers of her condition. Under the new notification procedures, it is unlikely that it would be necessary to notify any of her patients of the situation, since it is extremely unlikely that anyone has been infected. Brenda should discuss with her employers the possibility of her continuing to work in an area where there is minimal risk to any patients. Brenda should also be entitled for her identity not to made known in the press (see above).

Civil and criminal liability for endangering others

There would probably be civil liability if a health professional gave blood failing to disclose that he/she was a carrier of HIV/AIDS. If the health professional gave blood deliberately knowing that he/she could infect others, then as well as being a civil wrong under a principle established in an old 19th century case (*Wilkinson v. Downton* [1897]), the health professional could also be guilty of a criminal offence.

Stephen Kelly was convicted of knowingly infecting a lover with HIV and was jailed for five years (Harris 2001). He was prosecuted under the Scottish common law. The Criminal Injury Compensation Scheme recognises that a criminal offence leading to infection with HIV/AIDS should be compensated at level 17 of the tariff (currently £22000) (Criminal Injury Compensation Authority 2001).

In October 2003 Mohammed Dica was found guilty of inflicting biological bodily harm upon two lovers whom he had callously infected with HIV (Horsnell 2003). He was sentenced to eight years imprisonment, after the judge stated that his behaviour was despicable and he callously conned his victims into having unprotected sex with him. He appealed to the Court of Appeal and won a retrial on the grounds that the trial judge should not have withdrawn from the jury the issue of whether the women consented to intercourse knowing that he was HIV-positive (Ford 2004). In another case, an African who infected three women with

HIV after arriving in Britain as an asylum seeker was given a 10-year prison sentence (Norfolk 2004). The judge stated that the grievous bodily harm which he had inflicted on the women fell into the category of the very worst sort.

Protection of the health professional

A health professional who is HIV/AIDS-positive may have protection under the Disability Discrimination Act 1995, now reenacted in the Equality Act 2010 but the employer would be entitled to take reasonable measures to ensure that his/her patients were protected from the risk of cross-infection. There is no AIDS/HIV discrimination Act in the UK, so any employee suffering from AIDS or who was HIV-positive would have to claim protection from the Equality Act 2010 or other legislation including the statutory protection from unfair dismissal and the Human Rights Act 1998. To remedy the lack of protection for those who are HIV/AIDS sufferers, various organisations have published charters to protect their rights. For example, a charter was drawn up by some charities, including the Terence Higgins Trust (UK Declaration Working Group 1991). However, these charters do not in themselves have the force of law.

National strategy for sexual health and HIV services

In July 2001, the Department of Health announced a national strategy on sexual health and HIV services, aimed at preventing the spread of sexually transmitted diseases and at improving the care and treatment of those who need it, together with a new national information campaign to promote safe sex (Department of Health 2001). An independent advisory group (IAG) on sexual health and HIV was established in March 2003 (Department of Health 2003c) to monitor progress and advise the Government on the implementation of the Sexual Health and HIV Strategy. In January 2004 the IAG (Independent Advisory Group on Sexual Health and HIV 2004) responded to the Health Select Committees' Report on Sexual Health which was published in June 2003 (Health Select Committee 2003). The IAG welcomed the Government's emphasis on sexual health and HIV and agreed that there was much still to be done. In particular it agreed with the Select Committee's recognition of the six key factors which it believed were the principal causes of the current situation:

- A failure of local NHS organisations to recognise and deal with this major public health problem.

- A lack of political pressure and leadership over many years.
- The absence of a patient voice.
- A lack of resources.
- A lack of central direction to suggest that this is a key priority.
- An absence of performance management.

The IAG believed that sexual health and HIV must be explicitly prioritised at both a local and national level and as part of this prioritisation, allocated further resources to achieve the wholesale upgrading of services which is necessary to guarantee a significant improvement in sexual health in the country. In 2007, the Government commissioned the IAG to undertake a review of progress in implementing the 2001 sexual health and HIV strategy. The Department of Health (2009) published its response to this review in July 2009. This response set out the achievements in sexual health since 2001, and how the Government intended to implement the five priority areas identified by the IAG, i.e.:

- Prioritising sexual health as a key public health issue and sustaining high-level leadership at local, regional and national level.
- Building strategic partnerships.
- Commissioning for improved sexual health.
- Investing more in prevention.
- Delivering modern sexual health services.

The response is available on the Department of Health website.

Hepatitis

Guidance for hepatitis B infected workers was issued by the Department of Health in 2000 (Department of Health 2000). The guidance supplemented previous guidance (HSG (93)40 and EL(96) 77) restricting the working practices of certain hepatitis B-infected health care workers and aimed at reducing further the transmission of infection to patients. It recommended carrying out additional testing of hepatitis B-infected care workers who are e-antigen (HbeAG) negative and perform exposure prone procedures, and restricting the working practices of those with higher viral loads. More detailed guidance to assist in the implementation is available on the Department of Health website (www.dh.gov. uk/nhsexec/hepatitisb.htm).

As with a health professional suffering from HIV/AIDS there is a duty to inform the employer if the health professional becomes aware that they have hepatitis. A doctor who had been suspended by the General Medical Council (GMC) after he failed to inform his employers that he was suffering from a dangerous medical condition, lost his appeal in the High Court against his suspension. He was carrying hepatitis B and had not informed his employers even though he was carrying out exposure-prone procedures, including an open hernia repair (Nursing and Midwifery Council 2004). (For the compensation scheme for those infected with hepatitis C from blood products see *Chapter 12.*)

Following complaints by haemophiliacs that they were subjected to secret testing by doctors, the General Medical Council initiated an investigation in May 2003 to establish if the complaints were justified (English 2003).

Hepatitis C action plan

The Chief Medical Officer's infectious diseases strategy *Getting Ahead of the Curve* (2002) is considered in *Chapter 15.* The strategy was followed by a consultation on proposals to strengthen the services for prevention, diagnosis, and treatment and improve epidemiological surveillance and research. As part of the implementation of this strategy, the Chief Medical Officer of Health published an action plan for hepatitis C in June 2004 (Chief Medical Officer 2004). It estimated that there were approximately 200 000 people chronically infected in England and the majority were unaware of their infection.

There is currently no vaccine against hepatitis C, so prevention of new infections is particularly important. The action plan set out the framework of ongoing and new actions for the department, the NHS and other key stakeholders. It was designed to increase professional awareness of the disease and an information pack was being sent to primary care professionals. A website for professionals and the public has been created (www.hepc.nhs.uk) and a publicity campaign was launched in the autumn of 2004 to increase the awareness of hepatitis C and how to avoid the risk of infection, the testing for hepatitis C, and treatment. In 2006 the Health Protection Agency published standards for local surveillance and the follow up of hepatitis B and C, both acute and chronic. The foreword states that these standards were developed by a working party with wide representation across the Agency and they have been informed by consultation within the HPA and with a range of stakeholders. The standards recognise that the detection and clinical management of hepatitis B and C can involve a number of health professionals, creating a diversity of clinical pathways. The development of the standards has also taken into account the fact that the prevalence of both hepatitis B and C varies markedly across the country and that current systems for the surveillance and follow up of cases also vary. The Health Protection Agency publishes an annual report on Hepatitis C in the UK which is available on its website.

Conclusion

Contrary to some expectations, HIV/AIDS is continuing to be a growing concern in the UK and our laws relating to the rights of employees and patients are a patchwork of statutory and common law (judge-made law) provision. The Equality Act 2010 has brought together the laws relating to discrimination in a single statute and those who are HIV positive or have AIDS may find that they are protected against discrimination. The Health Protection Agency is a useful source of information on the topics considered in this chapter, but at the time of writing its future is in doubt as plans for a Public Health Service are due to be implemented.

References

Akinsanya J, Rouse P (1992) Who will care? A survey of the knowledge and attitudes of hospital nurses to people with HIV/AIDS. *Journal of Advanced Nursing* 17: 400–1

Baldwin T, Murray I (1999) All pregnant women must test for AIDS. *The Times* 13 August

Browne A (2002) Record HIV levels due to immigrants. *The Times* 30 November

Re C (HIV test) [1999] 2 FLR 1004 CA

Chief Medical Officer (2002) *Getting Ahead of the Curve: An infectious disease strategy.* Department of Health, London

Chief Medical Officer (2004) *The Hepatitis C Action Plan for England.* DoH, London

Criminal Injury Compensation Authority (2001) *Issue No 1 (4/01).* Home Office, London

Department of Health (1999 updated 2005) *AIDS/HIV Infected Health Care Workers: Guidance on the Management of Infected Health Care Workers and Patient Notification.* Department of Health, London

Department of Health (2000) *Hepatitis B Infected Health Care Workers: Guidance on implementation of Health Service Circular 2000/020.* Department of Health, London

Department of Health (2001) *National Strategy for Sexual Health and HIV Services.* Press release. Department of Health, London

Department of Health (2002) *NHS Update: New HIV Patient Information Policy.* Department of Health, London

Department of Health (2003a) *AIDS/HIV Infected Health Care Workers: Guidance on the Management of Infected Health Care Workers and Patient Notification.* Department of Health, London

Department of Health (2003b) *Health Clearance for Serious Communicable Diseases. New health care workers draft guidance for consultation*. Department of Health, London

Department of Health (2003c) *Health Minister Announces Group to Advise on Sexual Health*. Press release 6 March. Department of Health, London

Department of Health (2009) *Moving Forward: Progress and priorities – working together for high-quality sexual health - Government response to the Independent Advisory Group's review of the National Strategy for Sexual Health and HIV*. Department of Health, London

English S (2003) GMC to investigate 'secret testing'. *The Times*, 7 May

Ford RM (2004) Man who gave lovers HIV wins a retrial. *The Times*, 6 May

H (A healthcare worker) v. Associated Newspapers Ltd; H (A healthcare worker) v. N (A health authority) [2002] EWCA civ 195; [2002] Lloyds Law Rep Med 210; The Independent, 8 March

Harris G (2001) Five years for the reckless lover who passed on HIV. *The Times*, 17 March

Health Protection Agency (2006) *Standards for Local Surveillance and the Follow up of Hepatitis B and C* HPA, London

Health Protection (Notification) Regulations 2010 No. 659

Health Select Committee (2003) *House of Commons Select Committee Report on Health*. House of Commons, London: June

Henderson M (2003) Death toll from AIDS reaches 3 million a year. *The Times*, 26 November

Horsnell M (2003) Lover convicted after infecting women with HIV. *The Times*, 15 October

Independent Advisory Group on Sexual Health and HIV (2004) R*esponse to the Health Select Committee on Sexual Health*. January

NICE (2011a) *Guidance on Increasing the Uptake of HIV Testing Among Black Africans in England* Guidance no 33 NICE

NICE (2011b) *Guidance on Increasing the Uptake of Testing of Men who Have Sex with Men*. Guidance no 34 NICE

Nursing and Midwifery Council (2002) *Code of Practice. Rule 39*. NMC, London

Nursing and Midwifery Council (2004) *News Service*. 4 February. NMC, London

Norfolk A (2004) HIV man jailed for infecting women. *The Times*, 15 May

Royal College of Midwives (1998) *HIV and AIDS: Position Paper*. Royal College of Midwives, London

The Times (2004) News item: HIV needles alert. *The Times*, 4 December

United Kingdom Central Council for Nursing, Midwifery and Health Visiting (1992) *Anonymous testing for the prevalence of the human immunodeficiency virus (HIV)*.

Registrar's letter 8/1992, replacing circular PC/89/02 November. UKCC, London
UK Declaration Working Group (1991) Terence Higgins Trust, London
World Health Organisation (2011) *Fact sheet on HIV drug resistance* WHO
Wilkinson v. Downton [1897] 2 QB 57
X. v. Y. and Another [1988] 2 All ER 648

CHAPTER 17

Risk management

Scenario 17.1. An unreasonable instruction

Mammet, the manager of the podiatry department, was asked to carry out a risk assessment on health and safety. He had never been taught such an activity and needed to seek advice.

Introduction

Risk assessment and risk management is at the centre of health and safety in the work place and is a statutory duty set by the regulations on the management of health and safety in the workplace. This chapter considers the statutory duty and the guidance provided in relation to the Management of Health and Safety at Work Regulations 1999 and their relevance to the NHS. The management of risk is at the heart of health and safety laws. The law usually requires a risk to be managed 'so far as is reasonably practicable'. It does not place an absolute duty upon the employer to eradicate all risks from the workplace, but to take all reasonable measures to remove them or reduce the effect of their causing harm to employees and others. However, there are certain duties under health and safety legislation which are absolute: they have to be undertaken and there is no defence for a failure to carry them out (*Chapter 2*).

For example, in *Chapter 19* the regulations on manual handling are considered and it will be noted that whilst manual handling should be avoided, there is a qualification 'if it is reasonably practicable to do so'. This is not an absolute prohibition on manual handling but a requirement for the employer to take reasonable steps to prevent hazardous manual handling taking place. In contrast, there is an absolute duty to carry out a suitable and sufficient assessment where manual handling cannot be avoided. This duty has to be carried out and lack of resources, practicability problems and other such difficulties could not be used as a defence for failure to carry out a suitable and sufficient assessment. Similarly, under the Provision and Use of Work Equipment Regulations 1998 the courts have held that there is an absolute duty for work equipment to be maintained appropriately (*Chapter 2*).

Reasonable steps

Where a duty is 'reasonably practicable', it is for the employer to show that, taking into account the time, cost, practicality and other circumstances, it did what it reasonably could to avoid the manual handling. In the case of a prosecution brought by health and safety inspectors, it is for the prosecutors to show beyond reasonable doubt that an offence has been committed by the defendant. However, where the duty is one that should be performed so far as is 'reasonably practicable', then the defendant can attempt to prove on a balance of probabilities that it did all that was reasonably practicable to carry out the statutory duty. This is because it is within the knowledge of the defendant as to the reasonably practicable steps it took to comply with the duty. This defence will, therefore, involve reference to the records which were kept on the risk assessment and risk management. The defendant could also show that further costs were too high, or were not justified, or other circumstances made any further attempts to implement the reasonably practicable duty unreasonable.

The fact that a burden was placed upon a defendant under the Health and Safety at Work Act 1974 to establish on a balance of probabilities that he took all reasonably practicable steps was challenged in a case, as being in conflict with the Human Rights Convention Article 6(2) and the presumption of innocence (*Davies v. Health and Safety Executive* [2002]). However, the Court of Appeal held that the infringement of the presumption of innocence under Section 40 of the 1974 Act was justified and compatible with the Human Rights Act 1998.

Section 40 states that:

> *In any proceedings for an offence under any of the relevant statutory provisions consisting of a failure to comply with a duty or requirement to do something as far as it is practicable or so far as is reasonably practicable or to use the best means to do something that shall be for the accused to prove (as the case may be) that was not practicable or not reasonably practicable to do more than in fact was done to satisfy the duty or requirement or that there was no better practicable means than was in fact used to satisfy the duty or requirement.*

The Court of Appeal held that the 1974 Act was motivated by the need to protect public safety and the Act's regulatory nature meant that those operating within it had to conform to certain standards. In the field of health and safety it was acceptable to impose absolute duties on employers and it did not follow that a reverse burden of proof, within reasonable limits would infringe Article 6(2). The defendant was likely to have unique, special knowledge of the risk and the measures needed to avoid it. A merely evidential burden of proof may have led to the impossibility of enforcement given that the prosecution would have to go beyond showing the existence of a duty and prove what measures ought to have been taken.

Management of health and safety at work regulations 1999

These regulations were published in 1999 (Management of Health and Safety at Work Regulations, 1999) (revised since they were originally produced in 1992) and require employers to carry out a risk assessment. The Regulations are published with an approved code of practice and guidance (ACOP). The fundamental duty of the employer is shown in *Box 17.1*.

Box 17.1. Fundamental duty of the employer under the Management of Health and Safety at Work Regulations

Every employer shall make a suitable and sufficient assessment of the risks to the health and safety of his employees to which they are exposed whilst they are at work; and the risks to the health and safety of persons not in his employment arising out of or in connection with the conduct by him of his undertaking, for the purpose of identifying the measures he needs to take to comply with the requirements and prohibitions imposed upon him by or under the relevant statutory provisions and by Part II of the Fire Precautions (Workplace) Regulations 1997.

Guidance on risk assessment

The ACOP advises that a risk assessment should identify how the risks arise and how they impact upon those affected. This information is needed to make decisions on how to manage those risks so that the decisions are made in an informed, rational and structured manner, and the action taken is proportionate. Hazard and risk is defined in the ACOP as:

A hazard is something with the potential to cause harm (this can include articles, substances, plant or machines, methods of work, the working environment and other aspects of work organisation).

A risk is the likelihood of potential harm from that hazard being realised. The extent of the risk will depend on:

*   The likelihood of that harm arising.
*   The potential severity of that harm, i.e. of any resultant injury or adverse health effect.
*   The population which might be affected by the hazard, i.e. the number of people who might be exposed.

Realism of the risk assessment

The risk assessment must be a 'suitable and sufficient' assessment. These terms are not defined in the regulations, but the ACOP emphasises that the level of detail in the risk assessment must be proportionate to the risk. Once the risks are assessed and taken into account, insignificant risks can usually be ignored. In other situations, the risk assessment may need to be more sophisticated and specialist knowledge may have to be brought in. Employers will be expected to use all available information about the risks, e.g. relevant legislation, appropriate guidance, supplier manuals, manufacturers instructions, etc. The ACOP emphasises that there are no fixed rules about how a risk assessment should be carried out. Paragraph 18 of the ACOP suggests general principles that should be followed, and these are summarised in *Box 17.2*.

Box 17.2. Principles for a risk assessment

A risk assessment should:
*   Ensure the significant risks and hazards are addressed
*   Ensure all aspects of the work activity are reviewed, including routine and non-routine activities
*   Take account of non-routine operations, e.g. maintenance, cleaning operations
*   Take account of the management of incidents such as interruptions to the work activity
*   Be systematic in identifying hazards and looking at risks
*   Take account of the way in which work is organided and the effects this can have on health
*   Take account of risks to the public
*   Take account of the need to cover fire risks

Recording

Those employers with five or more employees must record the significant findings of their risk assessment. This record should represent an effective statement of hazards and risks which then leads management to take the relevant actions to protect health and safety. The record may be in writing or kept electronically. It must be retrievable by safety representatives, visiting inspectors and management as required (*Chapter 3*). The basic information which should be recorded is shown in *Box 17.3*.

Box 17.3. Recording a risk assessment

- A record of the preventative and protective measures in place to control the risks
- What further action, if any, needs to be taken to reduce the risk sufficiently
- Proof that a suitable and sufficient assessment has been made, with details of the assessment itself

---

Review and revision

Regulation 3(3) requires the employer to review the assessment if:

- There is reason to suspect that it is no longer valid.
- There has been a significant change in the matters to which it relates.

Where the review shows that changes to the assessment are required, there is duty on the employer to make these changes.

Preventive and protective measures

Regulation 4 requires employers to implement preventive and protective measures on the basis of the principles set out in schedule 1 of the regulations. These general principles of prevention (Council Directive 89/391/EEC OJ No L183, 29.6.89, p.1) can be seen in *Box 17.4*.

Box 17.4. General principles of prevention

- Avoiding risks
- Evaluating risks which cannot be avoided
- Combating risk at source
- Adapting the work to the individual
- Adapting to technical progress
- Replacing the dangerous by the non-dangerous or the less dangerous
- Developing a coherent overall prevention policy
- Giving collective protective measures priority over individual protective measures
- Giving appropriate instructions to employees.

Information to employees

Regulation 10 requires the employer to provide employees with comprehensible and relevant information of the risks to their health and the preventive and protective measures under Regulation 4.

Health and safety training

Regulation 13 requires employers to take into account the capabilities of employees as regards health and safety before entrusting tasks to them. The employer must ensure that employees are provided with adequate health and safety training when they are taken into employment and when they are exposed to new or increased risks. This training must be repeated periodically, where appropriate, adapted to take account of any new or increased risks, and must take place during working hours.

Duties of employees

Employees have a duty to use equipment in accordance with the training, and must inform the employer or any other employee with specific health and safety responsibilities of any work situation which represents a serious and immediate danger to health and safety, and any shortcomings in the employer's protection arrangements for health and safety.

Risk assessment and the NHS

The Clinical Negligence Scheme for NHS Trusts (CNST) requires trusts to undertake risk assessment and management in order to be members of the scheme in accordance with the standards set by the NHS LA (See *Chapter 18*). The visits of the CNST can be used by member trusts to establish their own standards of risk assessment and ensure that they are regularly monitored. Those NHS organisations who are not members of the CNST must ensure that they also comply with the legal requirements of the Management of Health and Safety at Work Regulations 1999.

Health and Safety Executive

Practical advice on reducing accidents at work is available from the Health and Safety Executive (HSE) and can be accessed through its website. In July 2003, the Chairman of the HSC wrote to all NHS chief executives highlighting the huge cost of accidents and work-related ill health to NHS staff and pointing out the benefits that proper management of these risks could bring, not only to staff, but also to the delivery of NHS services. His letter was sent in the light of the National Audit Office reports, *A Safer Place to Work: Improving the management of health and safety risks to staff in NHS trusts* (30 April 2003) and *A Safer Place to Work: Protecting NHS Hospital and Ambulance Staff from Violence and Aggression* (27 March 2003) (*Chapter 21*)

The five simple steps for risk management identified by the HSE are:

* Identify the hazards.
* Decide who might be harmed and how.
* Evaluate the risks and decide on precaution.
* Record your findings and implement them.
* Review your assessment and update if necessary.

The HSE emphasises the importance of not overcomplicating the process.

In many organisations, the risks are well known and the necessary control measures are easy to apply. You probably already know whether, for example, you have employees who move heavy loads and so could harm their backs, or where people are most likely to slip or trip. If so, check that you have taken reasonable precautions to avoid injury. If you run a small organisation and you are confident you understand what's involved, you can do the assessment yourself.You do not have to be a health and safety expert.

Application of the law to *Scenario 17.1*

It is unlikely that Mammet would be asked to undertake a risk assessment without having help and guidance. He should obtain a copy of the 1999 regulations referred to and seek the co-operation of the health and safety officer and his colleagues. The factors set out in *Box 17.2* would be a useful guide to follow. There are also advantages of linking a health and safety risk assessment with an assessment under the Control of Substances Hazardous to Health Regulations (*Chapter 10*). It is essential that a clear record should be made of the risks which are assessed and the action to be taken to remove or reduce those risks.

Conclusion

The management of risk is at the heart of health and safety laws. Risk assessment, therefore, must be carried out on a regular systematic basis across all activities within an organisation.

Records must be kept and action followed up and its success monitored. However it is essential that there is clear analysis of priorities in risk assessment. It was reported in one of the investigations into the BP oil disaster in the Gulf of Mexico that there were strict guidelines which barred BP employees from carrying a cup of coffee without a lid or walking down a staircase without holding a handrail, but there was no standard procedure for how to conduct a 'negative-pressure test' to avoid an oil well blow out (Frean 2011). All the HSE's publications on risk assessment emphasise the importance of giving attention to the most significant risks. Lord Young's report also wants industry to concentrate on real risks (see *Chapter 24*). Risk management is also an important activity within the concept of clinical governance, and it is to that which we turn in the next chapter.

References

Davies v. Health and Safety Executive [2002] EWCA Crim 2949 The Times 27 December 2002

Frean F (2011) BP 'took a harder line on coffee spills that the risk of a rig explosion'.
The Times 25 January 2011

Management of Health and Safety at Work Regulations (1999) Statutory Instrument 1999
No 3242. The Stationery Office, London

CHAPTER 18

Clinical governance

> ### Scenario 18.1. Risk assessment and tissuing
>
> Joshua worked in paediatrics and was concerned about the frequency of injuries caused to babies as a result of intravenous fluids being pumped into the tissue. It appeared that the mechanical pumps were not sufficiently sensitive to cut out when the vein tissued and there had been several cases where it appeared that serious harm had been caused to a baby.

Introduction

In *Chapter 7* we considered the statutory duty on the employer to undertake a risk assessment and management in relation to the health and safety of employees and others. In this chapter we consider the duty to assess and manage clinical risk. Risk management is seen as part of the concept of clinical governance. This will be explained and then the process of clinical risk management will be considered. In addition, the NHS organisation for inspection, the Care Quality Commission (CQC), will be discussed.

Clinical governance

The concept of clinical governance is based on the statutory duty of quality under Section 45 of the Health and Social Care (Community Health and Standards) Act 2003.

The duty of quality

The first statutory duty on the NHS to promote quality was contained in Section 18 of the Health Act 1999. This section has subsequently been amended by Section 11 of the NHS Reform and Healthcare Professions Act 2002 and then re-enacted in Section 45 of the Health and Social Care (Community Health and Standards) Act 2003 which states:

> *It is the duty of each NHS body to put and keep in place arrangements for the purpose of monitoring and improving the quality of health care provided by and for that body.*

Health care means 'the services provided to individuals for or in connection with the prevention, diagnosis or treatment of illness and the promotion and protection of public health'.

The duty to implement this falls primarily upon the chief executive of each health authority and NHS trust. In practice, each chief executive designates officers to be responsible for quality or clinical governance in specified areas of clinical practice. Government guidance was published in March 1999 (Health Service Circular 1999). This policy follows from the original consultation document *A First Class Service: Quality in the New NHS* (Health Service Circular 1998). The aim to develop quality within the NHS is to be secured in three ways:

- Setting clear national quality standards.
- Ensuring local delivery of high quality clinical services.
- Ensuring effective systems for monitoring the quality of services.

Risk management of clinical risks, therefore, depends upon the identification of risks, establishing standards of care to reduce those risks and setting up systems of audit and quality assurance to ensure that those standards are monitored. The main components of clinical governance are seen to be:

- Learning mechanisms (clinical risk management, clinical audit, adverse incident reporting, learning networks, continuing professional development).
- Patient empowerment (better information, patient complaints, patients' views sought and patients involved throughout the NHS).
- Knowledge management (information and information technology, research and development, education and training).

NAO progress report on clinical governance

In September 2003, the National Audit Office published a report on the implementation of clinical governance by NHS trusts. It concluded that progress in implementing 'clinical governance' is patchy, varying between and within NHS trusts and between components of the initiative. It stated that the structures and organisational arrangements to make clinical governance happen have been put in place in the corporate systems of most NHS trusts and the initiative has had many beneficial effects: clinical quality issues are now more mainstream and there is greater or more explicit accountability of both clinicians and managers for clinical performance. Reviews by the Commission for Health Improvement (replaced by the Commission for Healthcare Audit and Inspection and subsequently by CQC) have focused attention on improvements needed in individual trusts. The professional culture has also moved towards more open and collaborative ways of working.

However, the commitment to each component of clinical governance (such as clinical risk management, adverse incident reporting, better information for patients and use of information technology) within individual trusts varied widely. Clinical audit is not well established. Many trusts are not achieving effective standards of risk management.

The NAO recommended that the Department of Health should:

* Ensure that the Clinical Governance Support Team (part of the NHS Modernisation Agency) continues to develop and enhance its advice and support function, to satisfy the present unmet demand from trusts.
* Explore with the Clinical Governance Support Team more effective ways of disseminating good practice, including examples identified by the CHI (now CQC).
* Evaluate the impact of various patient empowerment initiatives and develop a set of good practice guidelines to help trusts make improvements in this area.

The NAO also recommended that NHS trusts should:

* Review the information requirements on quality issues required by their board and establish systems to ensure that such information is provided on a regular basis.
* Consider developing with their clinical teams systems of internal reporting on quality on the lines being developed by the Clinical Governance Support Team.
* Benchmark key clinical governance initiatives with similar trusts and build on and share examples of good practice.

Role of the Clinical Negligence Scheme for Trusts

The Clinical Negligence Scheme for Trusts (CNST) was established by the NHS Executive in 1994 to provide a means for trusts to fund the cost of clinical negligence litigation and to encourage and support effective management of claims and risk. The scheme covers claims arising from incidents on or after 1 April 1995. The NHS Litigation Authority (NHSLA), a special health authority, administers the scheme (see below). Membership is voluntary and open to all NHS trusts in England. Each trust can choose its own level of self-retention, and the scheme will contribute to the cost of claims in excess of this figure. Funding is on a 'pay as you go' non-profit basis. Actuaries appointed by the NHSLA analyse the available data and predict the total amount expected to be paid to the member trusts in respect of damages, costs and other expenses which will be incurred in the ensuing financial year. This amount is then apportioned between the member trusts. Individual trust contributions are based on a range of criteria, such as activities, budget, numbers of doctors by discipline, nurses and other professionals. These contributions can be reduced if a trust meets certain risk management criteria (initially the CNST risk management standards, now the NHSLA).

NHSLA standards and assessments

The NHSLA describes its standards and assessments in the following terms:

> *The core of our risk management programme is provided by a range of NHSLA standards and assessments. Most healthcare organisations are regularly assessed against these risk management standards which have been specifically developed to reflect issues which arise in the negligence claims reported to the NHSLA. There is a set of risk management standards for each type of healthcare organisation incorporating organisational, clinical, and health and safety risks: NHSLA Acute, PCT & Independent Sector Standards – 2010/11; NHSLA Mental Health and Learning Disability Standards – 2010/11; NHSLA Ambulance Standards – 2010/11. In addition, there is a separate set of clinical risk management standards for NHS maternity services. CNST Maternity Standards – 2010/11. NHS organisations which provide labour ward services are subject to assessment against both the NHSLA Acute (or PCT) Standards and CNST Maternity Standards.*

Manuals have been published containing the risk management standards for assessment from April 2011.

> *All the NHSLA Standards are divided into three 'levels': one, two and three. NHS organisations which achieve success at level one in the relevant standards receive a 10 percent discount on their CNST and Risk Pooling Schemes for Trusts*

(RPST) contributions, with discounts of 20 percent and 30 percent available to those passing the higher levels. The CNST Maternity Standards are also divided into three levels and organisations successful at assessment receive a discount of 10 percent, 20 percent or 30 percent from the maternity portion of their CNST contribution. Organisations at level 1 are assessed against the relevant standard(s) once every two years and those at levels 2 and 3 at least once in any three-year period, although organisations may request an earlier assessment if they wish to move up a level. Organisations at level 0 are assessed on an annual basis until such time as they achieve compliance. Organisations which fail an assessment are required to be assessed at the level assigned in the following financial year. All assessments take place over two days and are carried out on behalf of the NHSLA by Det Norske Veritas Ltd., who are responsible for much of the day-to-day administration of our risk management programmes. Details of the assessment levels achieved by health care organisations are updated monthly in our Factsheet 4.

Advice on the standards and general aspects of risk management is given in the NHSLA Review, and at workshops and seminars. The NHSLA has also created a number of template documents designed to assist organisations in developing their own local policies, procedures, etc. Use of these template documents is entirely optional. More template documents are to be introduced gradually over the next few years.

Clinical risk management and the NHS trust board

Risk management is a statutory duty to be carried out by every NHS and other health organisation. It has been defined as:

A means of reducing the risk of adverse events occurring in an organisation by systematically assessing, reviewing and then seeking ways to prevent their occurrence. Clinical risk management takes place in a clinical setting.

(NHS Executive 2001a)

Guidance has been provided by the NHS Executive on the topics which should be covered in the annual report to trust boards on clinical risk management (NHS Executive 2001a).

The guidance suggests that the four components of a risk management approach in a trust which require a critical assessment each year are:

- Is the right culture and risk management system being developed in the trust?
- What is going on now?
- What is its impact on patient care?
- Is it value for money?

The suggested contents of the annual report to the trust board are shown in *Box 18.1*.

A survey by the North Thames Region found that 90 percent of NHS trusts in the London region had introduced risk management, but only 56 percent had arranged specific training for staff and only 25 percent had provided a report for

---

Box 18.1. Contents of risk management report to trust board

1 Introduction
2 Structures
- *Staff support*
- *Clinical Claims Review Group*
- *Ad hoc investigation panels*
- *Risk Management Committee*
- *Local Risk Management Group*

3 Education and training for staff
4 Adverse Incident Reporting
- *Process and Database*
- *Overview of Data held on Database*
- *In-Depth Reviews: rolling programme*
- *Feedback of Incident Data*
- *Data Quality*

5 Links with Clinical Governance
- *Risk Management Involvement in other Corporate Groups*

6 Claims
- *Expert advice and support*
- *Claims profile CNST standards*
- *Clinical claims review group*

7 Improvements, new policies and actions
- *Risk management*
- *Complaints*

8 Costs
- *Staffing*
- *Claims/Legal/CNST costs*

9 Action Plan summary 2002/3
- *Future Development of Risk Management*
- *Current Position*

---

their board. In general practice, only 35 percent of practices had a health and safety manual (Department of Public Health and NHSE North Thames Region Office 1998).

In 2001, the NHS Executive published the results of a survey into the state of readiness of health authorities in London in undertaking risk management in primary care (NHS Executive 2001b). It appeared that at that time no health authority co-ordinated a programme of risk management in primary care. Since the survey, primary health care trusts have been given increased powers and there has been a reorganisation of health authorities to create strategic health authorities.

Care Quality Commission (CQC)

In accordance with the NHS Plan, the Health Act 1999 made provision for the establishment of a Commission for Health Improvement (CHI). Its main function was to ensure that standards are being maintained in the NHS. It fulfilled these by making regular inspections of NHS bodies and reporting to the Department of Health.

Under the Health and Social Care (Community Health and Standards) Act 2003, the CHI was abolished and replaced by the Commission for Healthcare Audit and Inspection (CHAI), with more extensive powers and duties. Following the Health and Social Care Act 2008 CHAI and other organisations, including the Mental Health Act Commission, were abolished and their functions were taken over by the Care Quality Commission in April 2009. The CQC is now the registration body and inspectorate for NHS and Independent hospitals, and adult social care providers. From October 2010, all adult social care and independent health care providers must be registered, with some exceptions (some providers of non-surgical laser and intense pulsed light services; domiciliary care agencies and nursing agencies that purely provide staff to other registered providers that do not arrange placements for people with personal care needs). From April 2011 the CQC registers primary care services that directly provide dentistry (NHS and private) and independent ambulance services. From April 2012, primary medical care services (including GP practices and out-of-hours services) must be registered. The CQC website provides information in relation to registration, compliance with its essential standards together with a directory of hospitals and care homes. Its website also contains the reports of individual inspections. Rules setting out the details of registration and the duties of the CQC are contained in the Regulations (Care Quality Commission (Registration) Regulations 2009/3112). The CQC published in guidance about compliance (CQC 2010). It has enhanced powers compared with its predecessor organisations in terms of the enforcement of its standards.

In the review of Arms' Length Bodies undertaken in 2010 (Department of Health 2010), no major changes were proposed in relation to the role of the CQC:

3.15 We therefore propose only limited changes to the Care Quality Commission's existing functions. The Care Quality Commission will continue to act as the quality inspectorate across health and social care for both publicly and privately funded care. To avoid double jeopardy and duplication, the NHS Commissioning Board will take over the current Care Quality Commission responsibility of assessing NHS commissioners, although the Care Quality Commission will continue to conduct periodic reviews of adult social care and retain its responsibilities under the Mental Health Act.

3.16 In relation to the NHS the Care Quality Commission will, together with Monitor (the regulator for NHS trusts), operate a joint licensing regime. The Care Quality Commission and Monitor already have a duty of co-operation in primary legislation to work closely together to ensure that the regulatory burden of multiple licences is reduced, whilst ensuring robust and proportionate regulation. In due course, subject to changes described elsewhere in this section, it is possible that the Care Quality Commission could take on responsibility for a broader range of licensing functions, including some of the functions of the Human Embryology and Fertilisation Authority and the Human Tissue Authority. Once again, we would expect to see a more integrated and coherent approach to licensing so that the outcome is effective and proportionate regulation, minimising the regulatory burden and maximising cost-effectiveness.

3.17 The Care Quality Commission will continue to inspect providers against essential levels of safety and quality in a targeted and risk-based way, taking into account information it receives about a provider. We intend that this information will come through a range of sources including patient feedback and complaints, Healthwatch England, GP consortia and the NHS Commissioning Board. Where inspection reveals that a provider is not meeting essential levels of safety and quality, the Care Quality Commission will take enforcement action to bring about improvement.

3.18 Finally, we propose that Healthwatch England, a new independent consumer champion, which will be an advocate for patients' rights and concerns, will be located with a distinct identity within the Care Quality Commission and will enjoy the benefits of the Care Quality Commission's independence and scale of operations, including avoiding duplicating work on the assessment of public opinions on health and care issues.

In April 2011 the CQC condemned the maternity department of Croydon University Hospital on the grounds that it was short on midwives and equipment and that training was not up to date and so women giving birth may not receive treatment from competent staff. Improvements had to be made within 28 days. Five mothers had died at the unit in 2010 and a report into the first three deaths found that one was avoidable and all involved poor care (*The Times* 2011)

Health Foundation

In 2011 the Health Foundation published its full report on research into the safety of clinical systems which showed serious deficiencies in the clinical information provided in outpatient clinics, prescribing for inpatients, handover in acute medicine, operating department equipment and the insertion of intravenous cannulae.

National Service Frameworks (NSFs)

The White Paper on the NHS (Department of Health 1997) set out a package of measures to raise standards within the NHS and these were further elaborated in the NHS Plan (Department of Health 2000). Included in this programme of action was the introduction of National Service Frameworks (NSFs). The circular (Health Service Circular 1998) explaining their function states:

> *NSFs will set national standards and define service models for a defined service or care group; put in place strategies to support implementation; and establish performance measures against which progress within an agreed timescale will be measured. The Commission for Health Improvement (CHI) will assure progress through a programme of systematic service reviews.*

Subsequently, NSFs have been prepared on the following topics:

* Cancer.
* Children.
* Coronary heart disease.
* Diabetes.
* Long-term health conditions.

- Mental health.
- Older people.
- Paediatric intensive care.
- Renal service.

Each NSF is developed with the assistance of an external reference group (ERG) which brings together health professionals, service users and carers, health service managers, partner agencies, and other advocates. External reference groups adopt an inclusive process to engage the full range of views. The Department of Health supports the ERGs and manages the overall process. In addition, the Department of Health makes a general invitation to professionals and the public to send in their views and their examples of good practice to the Department of Health website (www.dh.gov.uk).

The legal significance of NSFs

The NSF is not accompanied by statutory provision to enforce implementation, other than through the inspections of the CQC (an overview was originally provided by the NHS Modernisation Board and subsequently the NHS Quality Board). Guidance is issued by the Department of Health in the form of Health Service Circulars (HSCs) on implementation. For example, HSC 2001/026 sets out the standards defined in the NSF for diabetes (Health Service Circular 2001). Twelve standards are laid down from prevention of Type 2 diabetes to the detection and management of long-term complications. Standard 9 relates to diabetes and pregnancy. Failure by an NHS organisation to comply with the NSF could lead to a complaint by a patient but the patient could not sue for breach of a statutory duty since the NSF does not create statutory duties. If harm occurred to a patient and there was evidence that this harm resulted from a failure to follow a NSF, then a patient could argue that there was a failure to follow a reasonable standard of care. To succeed in this argument the patient would have to show that acceptable approved professional practice, as identified in the NSF, was part of what is known as the Bolam Test (*Bolam v. Friern HMC*). In addition, the patient would have to show that it was this failure to comply with the NSF which resulted in the harm for which he or she is seeking compensation. In theory therefore, a patient could sue if the NHS fails to provide services to the level set in the NSF, but only in the law of negligence and only if causation can be proved. Clearly, however, patients could use failures to provide minimum services as set out in an NSF as a basis of a complaint about the provision of services.

Statutory standards

In Section 46 of the Health and Social Care (Community Health and Standards) Act 2003 the Secretary of State has the power to set standards in health care which are legally binding upon health care providers. It would be possible for the Secretary of State in using the powers under Section 46 to create statutory duties for NHS organisations to implement NSFs.

National Institute for Health and Clinical Excellence (NICE)

NICE was established on 1 April 1999 to promote clinical excellence and cost-effectiveness (NICE 1999). The then Secretary of State stated that its task would be to abolish postcode variation in the country, so that there would be national standards for the provision of health care such as medicines. There had been a lack of uniformity in the decisions of health authorities over the provision of services, particularly of medicines. One of the functions of NICE is to issue clinical guidelines and clinical audit methodologies and information on good practice. NICE has a major role to play in the setting of standards of practice, by disseminating the results of research of what is proved to be clinically effective, research-based practice. It can be accessed on its website (www.nice.org.uk).

In November 2003, NICE published a consultation on a revised research and development strategy to strengthen guidance and improve the quality of patient care. The new strategy was finalised in May 2004. It is likely that eventually, as the guidelines of NICE become underpinned by more extensive research, there will be a presumption in favour of their being followed and the health professional would have to justify why in a particular situation NICE guidelines were not appropriate.

National Quality Board (NQB)

As part of the Darzi NHS reforms introduced by the Labour Government, an NHS Quality Board was established. The aim of the Board was to bring together all those with an interest in improving quality, to align and agree the NHS quality goals, whilst respecting the independent status of participating organisations. The Board's membership comprises a mix of skills and expertise and representation from some of the national statutory and professional bodies that make up the national quality landscape for health and social care. David Nicholson, the NHS Chief Executive, was chair of the Board. In addition, four members were appointed from within the Department of Health. They are: Sir Bruce Keogh, NHS Medical Director; Dame Christine Beasley, Chief Nursing Officer Sir Liam Donaldson, Chief Medical Officer; David Behan, Department of Health Director General for Social Care, Local Government and Care Partnerships. Four members were appointed from key national bodies with close links to the NHS: the Chair of the Care Quality Commission; the Chair of Monitor; the Chair of NICE and the Chair of the National Patient Safety Agency. In addition, approximately half of the NQB members have been appointed independently. The Appointments Commission has recruited expert and lay representatives from a broad variety of backgrounds, including professional bodies, frontline NHS staff, industry, universities, charities and international health care organisations.

The NQB held its first meeting on 30 March 2009, and produced an annual report on delivering quality in the Autumn of 2009 (NQB 2009).

On 17 March 2011 the NQB published its first report of a two-phase review of maintaining and improving quality during the modernisation of the NHS and beyond. The NQB outlines this as follows (NQB 2011a):

It describes the key roles and responsibilities of organisations and individuals that will protect and improve quality, suggests practical steps to safeguard quality during the transition; and emphasises the importance of the effective handover of knowledge and intelligence on quality between old and new organisations. The publication builds on the NQB's February 2010 'Review of Early Warning Systems in the NHS'. It emphasises how quality must remain the guiding principle as organisations move to implement the modernisation plans, and is clear that health care professionals are ultimately responsible for the quality of care provided to patients. This first report, 'Maintaining and Improving Quality during the Transition: Safety, effectiveness, experience', focuses on the first full year of transition 2011/12. Later in 2011 the NQB is to publish a further report with advice on how quality should be stitched into the fabric of the new architecture in order to maximise the potential for delivering high quality services for patients.

In addition, the NQB has published *Quality Governance in the NHS – A guide for provider boards* (NQB 2011b). This non-prescriptive tool can be used by provider boards to support organisations in ensuring resilience for quality.

The final report of the steering group for the national review of the hospital standardised mortality ratio (HSMR) has also been published. The steering group was established on behalf of the National Quality Board to review the methodology for calculating HSMR and recommend how these statistics should be used in the future.

Application of the law to *Scenario 18.1*

In theory, once an adverse incident takes place, lessons should be learnt, remedies implemented and such an incident should not reoccur. Joshua has a professional duty as a registered practitioner to take action to ensure that the lessons are learnt from these incidents and no more babies suffer such harm. He should, with colleagues, undertake a risk assessment to ensure that this particular risk is appropriately managed and does not occur again. For example, when the factors of this tissuing are analysed, it may be established that:

* The pumps which are being used for intravenous fluids are not appropriate for very young children.
* That when the cannula is set up there should be more frequent monitoring by nursing staff of the possibility of tissuing.
* That different times for monitoring should be set up when toxic substances are being infused.

Joshua should contact those managers in the hospital responsible for clinical risk management and clinical governance, and discuss how action can be taken to prevent this and other similar risks of harm. He should also check that the National Patient Safety Agency is contacted to ensure that they are notified of the incidents and that any research results or recommendations that they have published are obtained (*Chapter 13*). Notification should also be made to the Medicines and Healthcare Products Regulatory Agency (now performing the functions of the Medical Devices Agency) about failures in equipment (*Chapter 11*).

Conclusion

Clinical risk management should be an integral part of the work of every registered practitioner. In order for clinical governance to be successful it must become part of the culture and practice of each member of the organisation so that agreed standards for clinical practice are implemented and regularly monitored.

Ideally, a hazard should occur only once, lessons should be learnt from that incident, and action taken to prevent potential harm arising again. That is the function of the National Patient Safety Agency (*Chapter 13*). Every individual employee has a responsibility to learn the lessons and ensure that the appropriate action is taken.

References

Bolam v. Friern Hospital Management Committee [1957] 1 WLR 582

Care Quality Commission (2010) *Summary of Regulations, outcomes and judgement framework*. CQC, London

Department of Health (1997) *The New NHS — Modern, Dependable*. HMSO, London

Department of Health (2000) *The NHS Plan: A plan for investment, a plan for reform*. Cm 4818–1. Stationery Office, London

Department of Health (2010) *Liberating the NHS: Report of the Arm's Length Bodies*. HMSO, London

Department of Public Health, NHSE North Thames Region Office (1998) *Clinical Governance in North Thames: A Paper for Discussion and Consultation*. Department of Public Health, NHSE North Thames Region Office, London

Health Foundation (2011) *The Full Report Evidence: How Safe are Clinical Systems?* Health Foundation, London

Health Service Circular (1998) *A First Class Service: Quality in the New NHS*. NHS Executive, London

Health Service Circular (1999) *Clinical Governance: Quality in the New NHS*. NHS Executive, London

Health Service Circular HSC 1998/074 National Service Frameworks

Health Service Circular HSC 2001/026 Diabetes National Service Framework: Standards

National Audit Office (2003) *Achieving Improvements Through Clinical Governance: A progress report on the implementation by NHS trusts*. HC 1055 Session 2002–3. NAO, London

National Institute for Clinical Excellence (Establishment and Constitution) Regulations SI 1999 No 220; amendments SI 2002 No 1759 and 1760

National Quality Board (2009) *Delivering Quality*. Department of Health, London

National Quality Board (2011a) *Maintaining and Improving Quality During the Modernisation of the NHS and Beyond*. Part 1 2011-2012 DH 2011. Department of Health, London

National Quality Board (2011b) *Quality Governance in the NHS – A guide for provider boards*. Department of Health, London

NHS Executive (2001a) *Draft Template of Audit Risk Management Report for a Trust Board*. Department of Health, London (available from www.dh.gov.uk/london/clinicalgovernance/risktemp.htm)

NHS Executive (2001b) *Executive Clinical Governance in the London Region*. Department of Health, London

The Times (2011) Warning for maternity unit where five mothers died. *The Times* 28 April 2011

CHAPTER 19

Manual handling and repetitive strain injury

Scenario 19.1. A back injury

Poppy was a staff nurse on duty at night on an orthopaedic ward. Thomas, who had just been removed from traction, asked Poppy to assist him to go to the toilet. Poppy went to help him out of bed but, as she was helping him, she felt her back 'go' and cried out. She has subsequently been off work and is wondering about the legal situation.

Introduction

Back injuries have been a major cause of health problems for nurses and midwives. The Royal College of Nursing and the Royal College of Midwives have made strenuous efforts to ensure that their members are aware of the dangers in manual handling. Both colleges have supported members who have suffered back injuries from work in bringing civil cases for compensation. An important part of the case against employers is that there have been breaches of the health and safety regulations relating to manual handling. The HSE has provided guidance on the regulations as amended which was updated in 2004 (Manual Handling Operations Regulations 1992 (as amended); Guidance on Regulations L23 (Third edition) HSE 2004). It has also published a leaflet giving a concise practical guide to the law (*Getting to Grips with Manual Handling – A short guide*).

European directives on health and safety

In 1992, as a result of a European directive, the UK introduced six sets of regulations relating to health and safety (*Chapter 2*).

Manual Handling Operations Regulations 1992

Like the other regulations, the Manual Handling Operations Regulations 1992 (Statutory Instrument (SI) 1992 2793) came into force on 1 January 1993. They set very specific duties for the employer in relation to manual handling in the workplace. Amendments to the manual handling regulations were made by statutory instrument (Health and Safety (Miscellaneous Amendments) Regulations 2002 SI 2002 No 2174) which also gave effect to Council Directive 90/269 [1990] OJ L156/9 on the minimum health and safety requirements for the manual handling of loads where there is a risk particularly of back injury to workers. In respect of the amendment to the Manual Handling Operations Regulations 1992, Regulation 4 has been amended and is shown in *Box 19.1*.

Box 19.1. Amendments to manual handling regulations

In determining for the purposes of this regulation whether manual handling operations at work involve a risk of injury and in determining the appropriate steps to reduce that risk, regard shall be had in particular to::

a. The physical suitability of the employee to carry out the operations
b. The clothing, footwear or other personal effects he is wearing
c. His knowledge and training
d. The results of any risk assessment carried out pursuant to Regulation 3 of the Management of Health and Safety at Work Regulations 1999
e. Whether the employee is within a group of employees identified by that assessment as being especially at risk
f. The results of any health surveillance provided pursuant to Regulation 6 of the Management of Health and Safety at Work Regulations 1999

Manual handling operations are defined in the regulations as:

Any transporting or supporting of a load (including the lifting, putting down, pushing, pulling, carrying or moving thereof) by hand or by bodily force.

It can be seen from this definition that manual handling is a far wider concept than simply 'lifting' and that the actions set out in the brackets of the definition are only examples of manual handling operations. For example, catching is not actually mentioned, but this could come within the wider definition. Nor are there any exemptions from the definition of specialist forms of movement. Thus 'therapeutic lifting', when a patient is moved as part of therapy, would come within the definition of manual handling. The basic duties in relation to manual handling which are required by the manual handling regulations are given below.

Avoid hazardous manual handling if reasonably practicable

The first requirement is that manual handling, if hazardous, should be avoided if it is reasonably practicable so to do. This is not an absolute prohibition on manual handling, but a requirement for the employer to take reasonable steps to prevent hazardous manual handling taking place. It would be for the employer to show that, taking into account the time, cost, practicality and other circumstances, it did what it reasonably could to avoid the manual handling.

Make a suitable and sufficient assessment of any hazardous manual handling which cannot be avoided

The duty to carry out a suitable and sufficient assessment of any hazardous manual handling which cannot be avoided is an absolute duty. There can be no defence, for example, that an assessment was not reasonably practicable or too costly. Suitable and sufficient assessment has to be undertaken. Guidance is given in a schedule to the regulations on the factors which should be considered in relation to carrying out a suitable and sufficient assessment. The assessment should look at the tasks, the loads, the working environment and individual capability and various factors relating to these different aspects. In a case brought on the basis that there had been a breach of Regulation 4(b) of the Manual Handling Regulations 1992 and also a breach of Regulation 5 of the Provision and Use of Work Equipment Regulations 1992, a cleaner obtained compensation because of the failure of the employers to carry out a suitable and sufficient assessment of a new industrial quality vacuum cleaner and its failure to ensure that it was adapted to be suitable for the purpose for which it was to be used (*Watson v. Warwickshire CC* 2001).

Reduce the risk of injury from this handling so far as is reasonably practicable

Once the suitable and sufficient assessment has been carried out, action should be taken to implement the assessment in order to reduce, so far as is reasonably practicable, the risk of injury resulting from the manual handling.

Provide information about the load and centre of weight

The employer has a responsibility to give employees information about the weight of each load they are required to move and the heaviest side of any load whose centre of gravity is not positioned centrally. The regulations do not set a maximum weight to be lifted. In the view of the HSE:

> *The ergonomic approach shows clearly that such requirements (i.e. for maximum weights) are based on too simple a view of the problem and may lead to incorrect conclusions.*

Review the assessment

Any assessment must be reviewed if there are significant changes which make the original assessment inappropriate for the new circumstances. There is no time limit set for this review. The review would be required where there is reason to suspect that it is no longer valid or there has been a significant change in the manual handling operations to which it relates.

Duty of employee

Under Regulation 5 of the manual handling regulations each employee while at work must make full and proper use of any system of work provided for their use by their employer in compliance with the duty, set out under these regulations, to reduce the risk of injury from manual handling operations. This duty parallels the duty set out under Section 7 of the Health and Safety at Work Act 1974 on the employee to co-operate with the employer in the implementation of statutory duties and to take reasonable care of the health and safety of him/herself and his/her fellow employees (*Chapters 2 and 5*).

Lifting Operations and Lifting Equipment Regulations 1998 (LOLER 1998)

These regulations came into force for all lifting equipment on 5 December 1998, as a result of the lifting provisions of the Amending Directive to the Use of Work Equipment Directive (AUWED 95/63/EC). They are to be read in conjunction with the Provision and Use of Work Equipment Regulations 1998 (PUWER) (*Chapter 2*). They apply to all equipment including second-hand or leased equipment, and old and new equipment. The duty holders have to comply with all the requirements from 5 December 1998 (HSC 1998). Some of the pertinent LOLER regulations for health professionals are discussed below.

The definitions make it clear that 'lifting equipment' means work equipment for lifting or lowering loads and includes its attachments used for anchoring, fixing or supporting it. 'Load' includes a person. Paragraph 29 of the guidance on LOLER gives examples of the types of equipment and operations covered by the regulations and includes a bath hoist lifting a resident into a bath in a nursing home. Equipment used by many health professionals would therefore come within the regulations. Paragraph 47 of the guidance explains how the guidance applies to hoists:

> As hoists used to lift patients, e.g. from beds and baths, in hospitals and residential homes are provided for use at work and are lifting equipment to which LOLER applies, the duty holder, e.g. the NHS trust running the hospital or the owner of the residential home must satisfy their duties under LOLER.

In practice of course, the NHS trust would delegate the day-to-day responsibilities under the Regulations to the head of each clinical department.

Duties under the regulations include:

- Regulation 4: Every employer shall ensure that:
    (a) lifting equipment is of adequate strength and stability for each load, having regard in particular to the stress induced at its mounting or fixing point;
    (b) every part of a load and anything attached to it and used in lifting it is of adequate strength.

The Code of Practice paragraph 117 states that where the lifting equipment is used on rails it should be fitted with suitable devices; for example, to remove loose material from the rails to minimise the risks of the equipment being derailed.

- Regulation 5 covering lifting equipment used for lifting persons is set out in *Box 19.2*.
- Regulation 6 is set out in *Box 19.3*.
- Regulation 7 requires machinery and accessories for lifting loads to be clearly marked to indicate their safe working loads. Lifting equipment which is designed for lifting persons should be appropriately and clearly marked to this effect and lifting equipment which is not designed for lifting persons, but might in error be used for such a purpose, should be marked accordingly.

Box 19.2. Regulation 5 of LOLER

1. Every employer shall ensure that lifting equipment for lifting persons:
   (a) subject to sub para (b) is such as to prevent a person using it being crushed, trapped or struck or falling from the carrier;
   (b) is such as to prevent, so far as is reasonably practicable, a person using it, while carrying out activities from the carrier, being crushed, trapped or struck or falling from the carrier;
   (c) subject to paragraph (2) has suitable devices to prevent the risk of a carrier falling;
   (d) is such that a person trapped in any carrier is not thereby exposed to danger and can be freed
2. Every employer shall ensure that if the risk described in paragraph 1(c) cannot be prevented for reasons inherent in the site and height differences:
   (a) the carrier has an enhanced safety coefficient suspension rope or chain; and
   (b) the rope or chain is inspected by a competent person 'every working day'

Box 19.3. Regulation 6 of LOLER

1. Every employer shall ensure that lifting equipment is positioned or installed in such a way as to reduce as low as is reasonably practicable the risk:
   (a) of the equipment or a load striking a person; or
   (b) from a load:
       (i) drifting
       (ii) falling freely; or
       (iii) being released unintentionally; and is otherwise safe
2. Every employer shall ensure that there are suitable devices to prevent a person from falling down a shaft or hoist way

---

- Regulation 8 concerns the organisation of lifting operations and is set out in *Box 19.4*.
- Regulation 9 requires the employer to carry out a thorough examination and inspection before the equipment is first used unless it has not been used before and there is an EC declaration of conformity with the Lifts

---

Box 19.4. Regulation 8 of LOLER

1. Every employer shall ensure that every lifting operation involving lifting equipment is
(a) properly planned by a competent person;
(b) appropriately supervised; and
(c) carried out in a safe manner
2. In this regulation 'lifting operation' means an operation concerned with the lifting or lowering of a load

---

Regulations. The regulations require further inspections to be carried out at specified times.

- Regulation 10 provides for the person who makes the thorough inspection under Regulation 9 to notify the employer of any defect which, in his opinion, is or could become a danger to persons, sending a report to the enforcement agency if there is a risk of serious personal injury. Schedule 1 specifies the information which should be included in the report.
- Regulation 11 requires the employer to keep copies of reports of inspections and the time limits for which they should be held.

Enforcement of the regulations

Criminal prosecution

Like other statutory duties set out in health and safety legislation, the main agency for the enforcement of the manual handling and LOLER regulations is the Health and Safety Executive who, with its health and safety inspectors, has the responsibility for enforcement in the criminal courts (*Chapter 4*). In serious cases, individual employees could be prosecuted under Regulation 5 above. The most straightforward grounds for prosecution is where an employer has failed to carry out a suitable and sufficient assessment for manual handling, since this is an absolute offence, and no excuses could be used in defence by the employer. The absence of training of staff in risk management and manual handling operations could also be used as the basis, initially, of an enforcement notice and then if this was not complied with, by prosecution in the criminal courts.

Civil action

Civil action can be taken where an employee has been injured and it can be shown that there have been failures by the employer to provide the necessary training or hoists or staff for manual handling to be undertaken safely and that these failures have caused the harm suffered by the employee. In this case the employee may have a successful case against the employer for compensation for the harm which has been suffered (*Chapter 6*). The recent case of *Wiles v. Bedfordshire CC* is given in *Box 9.5*.

In another case, the Court of Appeal found in favour of an employee who had injured his back while carrying a microwave weighing between 15 and 20 kg (*O'Neil v. DSG Retail Ltd* 2002). The Court of Appeal found that:

- The employers had failed to assess the specific risk in relation to the particular task to be performed by the employee and was therefore in breach of the Manual Handling Regulations (Reg. 4(1)(b)(ii)).
- The employers had failed to take appropriate steps to reduce the risk by failing to give the training recognised as being necessary to increase awareness of the risk and reduce instinctive responses.

Box 19.5. *Case of Wiles v. Bedfordshire CC*

The County Court held that there was a breach of the Manual Handling Operations Regulations 1992 (Reg 4.1a) when 'W', a residential social worker, sustained an injury when taking a disabled girl, 'M', to the lavatory. W lifted the girl out of her wheelchair, propping her against the wall while she bent down to remove her underclothes, but the girl, whose upper limbs were prone to occasional involuntary spasms, threw out her hands and fell backwards on to W, who suffered a back injury.

W claimed that two persons should have carried out that activity. Following the incident, staff were instructed to use a hoist and two staff when taking M to the lavatory. The judge held that even though at the precise time W was not actually carrying out a manual handling operation, the whole task of taking M to the lavatory should be considered a manual handling operation. The employers were in breach of the regulations by failing to avoid the need for manual handling and for failing to carry out a proper assessment or taking steps to reduce the risk of injury.

- It was reasonably foreseeable that an employee would twist whilst supporting a load.
- Failure to provide the appropriate training was therefore, on the balance of probabilities, a cause of the accident.

Ambulance technician and manual handling

The microwave case contrasts with another decision of the Court of Appeal in another manual handling case (*King v. Sussex Ambulance NHS Trust* [2002]) where the Court held that the employers were not in breach of the directive or regulations on manual handling. King, an ambulance technician, suffered serious injuries carrying an elderly patient down the stairway of his home. He and his colleague had taken the patient down the stairway, which was narrow and steep, in a carry chair. He had been injured when forced for a brief moment to bear the full weight of the chair.

The judge found in favour of the ambulance technician holding that the employers were in breach of Council Directive (90/269; Article 3(2)) and the Manual Handling Regulations, and that the employers had acted negligently by discouraging employees in circumstances, such as those in this particular case, from calling the fire brigade to take patients from their homes.

Sussex Ambulance NHS Trust appealed against the finding. The Court of Appeal held that the NHS trust was not liable either under the Directive or under the Manual Handling Regulations. There was nothing to suggest that calling the fire brigade would have been appropriate in the case. The evidence showed that such an option was rarely used because it had to be carefully planned, took a long time and caused distress to the patient. There might be cases where calling the fire brigade would be appropriate, but that would depend on the seriousness of the problem, the urgency of the case, and the actual or likely response of the patient or his/her carers and the fire brigade.

King had failed to show that giving that possibility more emphasis in training would have avoided his injuries. The ambulance service owed the same duty of care to its employees as did any other employer. However, the question of what was reasonable for it to do might have to be judged in the light of its duties to the public and the resources available to it when performing those duties. While the risks to King had not been negligible, the task that he had been carrying out was of considerable social utility.

Furthermore, Sussex Ambulance NHS Trust had limited resources so far as equipment was concerned. There was no evidence of any steps that the trust could have taken to prevent the risk and the only suggestion made was that it should have called on a third party to perform the task for it. Since calling the fire brigade was not appropriate or reasonably practicable for the purpose of the directive and the regulations, the Sussex Ambulance NHS Trust had not shown a lack of reasonable care. Accordingly, it had not acted negligently.

In contrast to the ambulance case, a nurse aged 36 years was awarded £420000 in damages by the High Court for a crippling back injury caused by her lifting a patient at Newham General Hospital, East London (*The Times* 2002).

These cases show that each case depends upon the facts and what can be established before the court. Records of risk assessments and decisions on risk management and the evidence of witnesses as to what had taken place are crucial in determining whether the employee obtains compensation.

A former nurse was awarded £47 621 plus legal costs for an injury that occurred nine years before. She was helping an elderly woman to use a commode at her home when the injury occurred. She was using a method of rocking the patient from side to side to help her adjust her clothes. The injury accelerated a pre-existing spine condition by about five years, rendering Mrs Rowe unfit for work. She told the court that she had been instructed to use the method by her NHS trust and had done so several times without realising it was dangerous to herself. The judge found the NHS trust liable because it had instructed her to use an unsafe procedure while tending to a patient and rejected the trust's arguments that Mrs Rowe, a nurse with 30 years' experience, should have been aware of the dangers. The judge held that there was no contributory negligence (NMC News 2003).

Accident and Emergency Nurse (*Postle v. Norfolk and Norwich NHS Healthcare Trust* 2000)

Mr Postle was employed as a nurse in the accident and emergency department when a patient collapsed in the waiting area and was placed on a hospital trolley. He was standing by the right side of the trolley towards the foot, but was not actually holding or pulling it. Another nurse, A, pulled the trolley from the front and towards the left, so that the rear of the trolley swung to the right and struck Postle thereby causing him a back injury. He claimed damages for negligence and for breach of statutory duty, namely the Manual Handling Operations Regulations 1992 Reg. 4(1)(b)(ii). The defendant NHS trust claimed that the Regulations were inapplicable because the duty imposed by them on the employer was owed only to an employee who was carrying out an operation in respect of injuries which he or she may suffer whilst doing so and in the instant case they could not be invoked by the claimant because the manual handling operation was being carried out by another nurse, A, and not the claimant. The claimant lost his claim for compensation. The judge held that the Regulations were applicable: they should not be read in a restrictive sense, but should apply to the whole of what was essentially a single operation. However, the defendant health trust was not in breach of the Regulations: a suitable and sufficient assessment would not have recognised the risk of injury to one nurse from the pulling of a trolley by another, nor would steps to reduce the risk have involved giving instructions which should have led A to pull the trolley forward, rather than to the left, or to tell the other nurses that she was about to move.

Contributory negligence

In some cases the amount of compensation which a claimant can obtain will be reduced to take account of that person's fault in causing the injury. For example, in a case in 1997 (*McCaffery v. Datta* [1997]) a nurse was held to be one-third contributorily negligent for her back injury because she had a previous injury to her back and was given medical advice not to undertake heavy lifting work, but she had not arranged the patient's bed so as to maximise the best way of lifting. Her appeal to the Court of Appeal failed, since it was held that there was ample evidence to support the finding of contributory negligence (*Chapter 5*).

Manual handling and human rights

In *Box 19.6* the tragic case of Mr and Mrs Bouldstridge is set out. The judge was not required to decide if requiring a client to use a hoist is contrary to the human rights of the client.

In another newspaper report of the case (Paul Kelso), the background facts were set out more fully. Here it explained that his wife had, over six years, gradually deteriorated to the point, where doubly incontinent and completely immobile she required assistance from two carers three times a day, seven days a week. In March, Mr B was informed by Hampshire Social Services that unless he had a hoist installed to help lift his wife, her carers would be withdrawn. On 11 March her carers had refused to lift her manually leaving him unable to feed or clean his wife. *The Guardian* reports that, 'his fear that she would be left without sufficient care was the straw that broke the camel's back. Distraught with anxiety and out of his mind, he decided to end his wife's suffering and his own.' Mr B had written a note blaming a social worker and the owner of the private care company, claiming that the fear that his wife would be left unattended drove him to do what he did.

Box 19.6. The Bouldstridge case (Johnstone 2000)

A pensioner of 84 was prosecuted after he had attached a length of hose pipe to the exhaust of his car and fed it into the home of himself and his wife. He joined his wife in the bedroom, leaving a suicide note, but a neighbour switched off the car engine and alerted the emergency services. The wife died in a nursing home the next month after developing an unrelated chest infection. The wife had Alzheimer's disease and her husband was unable to communicate with her. The judge criticised the prosecution for bringing the case and said that he was satisfied that, 'you were the victim of cruel and longstanding circumstances. You found yourself at your wits' end and did something which was morally indefensible, although humanly very understandable'. He was sentenced to probation of a year after he had pleaded guilty to the attempted murder of his wife.

Comments on the Bouldstridge case

Whilst one can have every sympathy with Mr Bouldstridge and his wife, *The Guardian* report does not give any details from the social services and private care company perspective. Why did Mr B not want the hoist to be used? Had it been delivered? Had he seen it in use elsewhere? Had he been advised that if he was not prepared to allow the hoist to be used, his wife would have to be cared for in residential accommodation? This would in practice seem to be a better alternative than to simply leave him on his own without any carers coming to visit her. Clearly, we do not have all the facts of this case and the *Guardian* write up seems extremely harsh on the social services, who may have other extremely relevant information which was never made public. Alternative action which social services could have taken was to apply to court for a direction as to the entitlement to insist upon the use of a hoist as an alternative to residential care. However, they probably had no idea of the lengths to which Mr B would go in his frustration.

East Sussex case

In a case in East Sussex (*Box 19.7*) where clients objected to the use of hoists, the judge emphasised that it was for the authority to carry out a risk assessment for manual handling and not for the court. The judge refused to state that there was a human right not to be hoisted, nor did he state that the care assistants had

---

Box 19.7. *A and B v. East Sussex County Council* [2003]

A and B were sisters, 26 and 22 at the time of the hearing, who both suffered from profound physical and learning disabilities and who had always lived in the family home, which had to an extent been specially adapted and equipped for them. They were looked after on a full-time basis by their mother and stepfather. They both suffered from greatly impaired mobility. Even the simplest physical movement, for example, getting out of bed or getting into a bath, required them to be moved and lifted by their carer. East Sussex provided services to them under section 2 of the Chronically Sick and Disabled Persons Act 1970, section 29 of the National Assistance Act 1948 and section 47 of the NHS and Community Care Act 1990. Central to the disputes which had arisen between the family and East Sussex Council was the extent to which the necessary moving and lifting should be done manually or by the use of appropriate equipment.

---

a human right to insist on a hoist being used. He stated that whether hoisting was appropriate would depend upon the actual circumstances of the case (*A and B v. East Sussex County Council*).

In his judgment in the case of A and B against East Sussex Council, the Hon Mr Justice Munby explored statutory provisions relating to manual handling, case law, the articles of the European Convention on Human Rights and case law on the interpretation of the articles. He accepted that both A and B and also their carers had rights under Article 8 of the European Convention on Human Rights to dignity. He stated it was highly questionable to state that manual handling is dignified whereas mechanical handling is undignified and said:

One must guard against jumping too readily to the conclusion that manual handling is necessarily more dignified than the use of equipment... Hoisting is not inherently undignified, let alone inherently inhuman or degrading. I agree... that certain forms of manual lift, for example the drag lift, may in certain circumstances be less dignified than hoisting. Hoisting can facilitate dignity, comfort, safety and independence. It all depends on the context.

The judge went on to consider a framework for decision making, setting out the principles which should apply and considering the factors which should be taken into account in determining how to assess reasonable practicability. These factors included:

- The possible methods.
- The context.
- The risks to the employee.
- The impact upon the disabled person which would necessitate an analysis of her physical and mental personality; their wishes and feelings; effect upon the person's dignity and rights.

Following this assessment, there then had to be a balancing exercise between the assessment of the carer and of the disabled person. Once the balance has been struck, if it comes down in favour of manual handling, then the employer must make appropriate assessments and take all appropriate steps to minimise the risks that exist. The assessment must be properly documented and lead to clear protocols which cover *all* situations, including foreseeable emergencies and, in the case of patients such as A and B, events such as spasm and distress which might arise. The outcome of the case was that the judge required East Sussex to carry out the necessary assessments for each activity for A and B, taking into account the considerations and factors which he had set out.

In another case it was reported in a news item (*The Times* 2003) that a disabled woman who had had to sleep in a wheelchair for 17 months after nurses stopped lifting her in case they were injured, could soon be able to use her own bed again. A High Court judge ordered that arrangements for moving Lorraine Wolstenholme, aged 50 years, from Milton Keynes, be made. In a case in 2008 (reported by Workplace Law Network) a care assistant who was injured while lifting a patient was awarded £8000. She injured her back whilst lifting a resident at The Grange Residential Care Home in Darlington.

An example of a prosecution under LOLER regulations

A Liverpool nursing home was fined £18000 after an 81-year-old woman fell to the ground while being lifted out of bed. Frances Shannon fell three feet and suffered a broken shoulder as well as injuries to her back and elbow. The wife, mother of two and grandmother of one, died in the Royal Liverpool University Hospital the following day. The Catholic Blind Institute, which runs the Christopher Grange nursing home, was prosecuted by the Health and Safety Executive (HSE) for failing to carry out regular checks of the lifting sling being used. It pleaded guilty to the offence and was sentenced at Liverpool Crown Court on 17 January 2011. The court heard that Mrs Shannon was being moved from her bed to a wheelchair at the Christopher Grange Nursing Home, on Youens Way in Knotty Ash, on 4 December 2008 when the sling failed.

Sarah Wadham, the investigating inspector at the HSE, said:

> Mrs Shannon's fall would have been prevented if the Catholic Blind Institute had complied with the law for using equipment to lift people. There should have been regular checks of the sling and it should have been thoroughly examined at least once every six months. Sadly this did not happen. I would urge care providers, including NHS trusts, primary care trusts and care homes, to ensure that they carry out the necessary examinations and inspections of lifting equipment, to prevent similar tragic incidents in the future.

The Catholic Blind Institute was charged with breaching Regulation 9(3) of the Lifting Operations and Lifting Equipment Regulations 1998. It was ordered to pay £13876 towards the cost of the prosecution in addition to the fine.

Regulation 9(3) of the Lifting Operations and Lifting Equipment Regulations 1998 states:

> Every employer shall ensure that lifting equipment which is exposed to conditions causing deterioration which is liable to result in dangerous situations is thoroughly examined in the case of lifting equipment for lifting persons or an accessory for lifting, at least every 6 months...and if appropriate for the purpose, is inspected by a competent person at suitable intervals between thorough examinations, to ensure that health and safety conditions are maintained and that any deterioration can be detected and remedied in good time.

HSE guidance on manual handling

In August 2003, the HSE published a manual handling assessment chart (MAC) and also set up a website (www.hse.gov.uk/msd/mac) which can be used by employers, employees, safety representatives and others to obtain information about, case studies of, and guidance and research on musculoskeletal disorders. The MAC is designed to help make easy and accurate assessments of three different types of operation: lifting, carrying and team handling. It records risk factors and provides a risk rating: green, amber, red or purple on a score sheet. The HSE has also published answers to frequently asked questions which include advice on team handling. Many leaflets prepared by the HSE on manual handling are available from its website. It has also published several case studies on practical means of avoiding some of the risks inherent in manual handling an example of which is shown in *Box 19.8*.

Box 19.8. HSE case study on manual handling

Mr G had multiple sclerosis and was cared for by two workers. He had full use of his arms and hands but little strength in his legs and feet. He weighed 12 stone/75kg. The care workers would wash Mr G while he was in bed. One care worker would roll Mr G towards her and the second would wash his back. The holding task was uncomfortable for the worker and caused lower back pain. The occupational therapist reviewed the risk assessment and identified the holding task as a manual handling risk.

An Action Bed rail was used to make use of patient strength. To make best use of Mr G's arm strength, bed rails were installed which were screwed to the floor and were above the height of the bed. This allowed Mr G to reach across with his opposite arm and use the rails to roll and support himself in that position. The cost of the bed rails was £70 and installation was £40.

This action was beneficial because it reduced the manual handling risk to the care workers. Using the strength in his arms helped Mr G to maintain mobility and feel less dependent. He liked being able to assist his care workers.

(HSE 2002)

Application of the law to *Scenario 19.1*

In order to determine whether Poppy would have a case for compensation, it is necessary to have more facts:

- Has Poppy been trained in risk assessment and manual handling?
- Has a risk assessment of manual handling for Thomas been undertaken following his removal from traction?
- Are there any instructions which Poppy has failed to carry out in relation to the early ambulation of Thomas?
- Does the assessment indicate that a hoist should have been used?

If from such information it is possible to show that there has been a failure by the NHS trust to comply with the manual handling regulations, and as a consequence Poppy has injured her back, then she may be able to claim compensation from her employer. If she has failed to implement the principles which she has been trained in, there may be evidence of contributory negligence, and this would mean that her compensation would be reduced accordingly.

Repetitive strain injury (RSI)

Scenario 19.2. Too much typing?

Florrie was a typist in the medical secretaries typing pool at Roger Park Hospital NHS Trust and complained that at night she suffered shooting pains up her arm and her wrist which were extremely painful. She sought medical advice and was told that she should try and avoid work on a keyboard for several months. She notified the trust who told her that it was not possible to offer her any suitable alternative work and if she could not continue her duties they would consider her to have resigned. She is now seeking legal advice to find out if she could sue the trust for the loss of her job and for compensation for repetitive strain injury.

Even though in an early case, a judge was quoted out of context as declaring that repetitive strain injury (RSI) has no place in medical books (*Mughal v. Reuters Ltd* 1993), RSI has been recognised for the purpose of compensation in health and safety cases. In the case of *Bettany v. Royal Doulton UK Ltd* the High Court found that repetitive work causing only pain with no other associated symptoms could be classed as an overuse injury caused by the plaintiff's work, but on the actual facts of the case, the employers were not found to be in breach of the duty of care which they owed to the employees (the employers had warned her of the dangers, had introduced a system of reporting problems and had moved her to lighter work). The HSE has estimated that in 2005/06 about 374 000 people in Great Britain suffered from an upper limb disorder (ULD) caused or made worse by their work. It states that

> ULDs can result from various kinds of work. On the HSE website can be found information of use to employers, workers, occupational health professionals or those just interested in the treatment and management of ULDs. ULDs can be associated with the use of display screen equipment (DSE) or work using vibrating tools.

A decision of the House of Lords, however, may make it more difficult to obtain compensation for RSI or ULD (see *Box 19.9*).

The House of Lords held that the Court of Appeal should not have overruled the findings of the High Court Judge, since he had ample evidence before him to justify his decision that in the plaintiff's case the giving of warnings was unnecessary, even though typists in another department had been given warnings.

In an RSI case involving an industrial radiographer, the radiographer was successful in claiming compensation (*Hunter v. Clyde Shaw Plc*). Hunter was

---

Box 19.9. RSI claim rejected (*Pickford v. ICI*)

On 25 June 1998 the House of Lords rejected claims that a secretary who was sacked after she developed a form of repetitive strain injury should be able to sue her employers. It overruled the Court of Appeal decision that Ann Pickford should be allowed to make a claim against Imperial Chemical Industries. The Court of Appeal had found that ICI was negligent in failing to warn her of the need to take breaks during her work using a word processor and gave her the right to take her case back to the High Court for an assessment of damages, which she estimated at £175000. In a majority judgment (4 to 1) the House of Lords decided that ICI did not need to warn her about the dangers of repetitive strain injury, because typing took up only a maximum 75 percent of her workload.

To impose a warning which might cause more harm than good would be undesirable, since it might be counter-productive. The House of Lords questioned whether she had proved that the pain was organic in origin. She had been sacked in 1990 after taking long periods off work because of pain in both hands. She claimed that the injury had been caused by the very large amount of typing at speed for long periods without breaks or rest periods. The House of Lords said that it could reasonably have been expected that a person of her intelligence and experience would take rest pauses without being told. It also held that RSI as a medical term was unhelpful. It covered so many conditions that it was of no diagnostic value as a disease. PDA4 (Prescribed disease A4) had, however, a recognised place in the Department of Health and Social Security's list for the purposes of industrial injury, meaning a cramp of the hand or forearm due to repetitive movements such as those used in any occupation involving prolonged periods of handwriting or typing.

---

an industrial radiographer aged 48 years who suffered from lateral epicondylitis (tennis elbow) from moving castings, mainly of between one and five tonnes on a turntable at work. Although he complained of pain in his right arm in late 1990, he was left to operate the turntable alone from March 1991 until he ceased work and consulted a doctor for pains in his arm in June 1991. He was made redundant in December 1991. As a result of operations to his left arm in October 1992 and his right arm in March 1993, he was left with weakness and pain on squeezing and gripping both arms. His ability to garden, drive and write were impeded and he was unable to assist his wife with lifting and shopping. His ability to play darts and bowls were also restricted. An expert hand surgeon stated for the defendants that it was not scientific to assert that this tennis elbow was work related as the condition arose constitutionally but could be aggravated externally. His claim succeeded and he was awarded £8000.

Ian Arrowsmith analysed the reasons why radiographers suffer work-related upper limb disorders (Arrowsmith 2001). He concluded that over 70 percent of radiographers, responding to his study, suffered work-related upper limb disorders (WRULD) and that the demographic factor which has most effect on the likelihood of suffering from such a disorder was age, with those over 36 years most likely to experience the symptoms. The working conditions likely to produce WRULD are heavy workload, poor equipment design, lack of training and awareness of both staff and management. All these are factors which could be overcome. David Chapman-Jones analysed the problem of musculo-skeletal injury (MSI) for sonographers (Chapman-Jones 2001) and concluded that existing research of the incidence of MSI did not take account of their out-of-work lifestyles and there was probably a lower incidence which was directly attributable to the work of sonographers. He did consider that, 'the symptoms that the sonographers are presenting with could be reduced or eliminated if working practices, primarily, and lifestyle are modified to accommodate such diversion from our natural state'. He recommended that there should be serious review of working practices to avoid a flood of occupational-induced musculo-skeletal disorder compensatory claims.

RSI and back injury

It was reported in *The Guardian* in 2001 that a former staff nurse, Carmel Commons, received compensation for £345000 for back pain she suffered as a result of working at the Queen's Medical Centre, Nottingham, which allegedly lacked the correct equipment to move patients. She is the first nurse to have won a case involving repetitive strain rather than injury from a single incident.

Application of the law to *Scenario 19.2*

Florrie has several different claims. The success of her claim for compensation for personal injury from the employers will depend upon her being able to prove that she was suffering from a work-related disorder, that a reasonable employer would have foreseen the possibility of her suffering from this condition as a result of her working conditions, that there were reasonable steps which the employer could have taken, and that her employer failed to take these steps. (For example, it may have been possible to alternate her keyboard work with other work such as filing, or other administrative work). The burden is on Florrie to prove, on a balance of probabilities, the breach of duty by the employer that this caused the harm that she suffered and that her injury is significant (see *Chapter 5*). She also may have a claim for constructive dismissal, by showing before an employment tribunal that her employers were in fundamental breach of contract when they failed to provide alternative work for her and to take account of the risks to her health by working constantly at the keyboard. If she can establish constructive dismissal in this way, then the employers would have to show that the dismissal was fair, which would be extremely difficult.

Conclusion

All health practitioners are required in law to understand the implication of the manual handling and lifting regulations, and ensure that they have the requisite training. Clearly, it is essential that documentation relating to training in manual handling and the records of risk assessments on manual handling are kept since they will be important evidence in any dispute. Any health service employer should also carry out a risk assessment of the possibility of an employee suffering from RSI or WRULD, and ensure that all reasonable steps are taken to reduce any such reasonably foreseeable risk. Again documentation of the risk assessment and the action taken is essential.

References

A and B v. East Sussex County Council (The Disability Rights Commission an interested party) [2003] EWHC 167 (Admin)

Arrowsmith I (2001) Why do radiographers suffer work-related upper limb disorders? *Synergy* March: 6–9

Bettany v. Royal Doulton UK Ltd reported in Health and Safety Information Bulletin

1994 'Unidentifiable ULD/RSI can be occupationally caused' HSIB 219 20

Chapman-Jones D (2001) Musculo-skeletal injury: Is it a problem for sonographers? *Synergy* April: 14–15

Guardian (2000) Paul Kelso He only wanted to end his wife's pain. *Guardian* 7 June

Guardian (2001) News item. *Guardian* 6 June: 6

HSC (1998) *Safe Use of Lifting Equipment. Approved Code of Practice and Guidance.* Health and Safety Executive books, London

HSE (2002) *Handling Home Care: Achieving safe, efficient and practical outcomes for care workers and clients.* HSG225 HSE Books, London

HSE (2004) *Guidance on Regulations L23* (Third edition) HSE Books, London

Hunter v. Clyde Shaw Plc [1995] SLT 474;[1994] SCLR 1120

Johnstone H (2000) Man, 84 tried to kill sick wife. *The Times* 7 June

King v. Sussex Ambulance NHS Trust [2002] EWCA 953; Current law August 2002 408

McCaffery v. Datta [1997] P.I.Q.R. 64

Mughal v. Reuters Ltd [1993] IRLR 571

NMC News (2003) Unsafe procedure led to injury. *NMC News*: 29 October

O'Neil v. DSG Retail Ltd 2002 The Times 9 September; Current Law October 2002 209

Pickford v. Imperial Chemical Industries Plc The Times Law Report 30 June 1998 HL [1998] 1 WLR 1181

Postle v Norfolk and Norwich NHS Healthcare Trust September 19 2000 County Court (Current Law 2000 2970)

The Times (2002) News item: £420000 award. *The Times* 17 October

The Times (2003) News item: Date for moving. *The Times* 19 November

Watson v. Warwickshire CC (2001) Current Law October 284

Wiles v. Bedfordshire CC CLR (2001) 365 June

CHAPTER 20

Stress and bullying

Scenario 20.1. Stress at work

Iris works in the intensive care unit at Roger Park Hospital. One of her responsibilities is to arrange the rota for staff cover. As a result of the shortage of intensive care nurses locally, she is compelled to use agency nurses and to plead with her colleagues to work additional shifts or overtime. On some occasions she has been close to asking senior management to consider halting admissions and leaving beds empty, because she is unable to arrange cover. She increasingly finds that she is unable to cope with the situation: she is unable to sleep, she is worrying about work when not on duty and feels that she is close to a nervous breakdown. What is the law?

Introduction

Concern with stress at work is now recognised as part of the employer's duty in taking reasonable care of the health and safety of the employee. One of the first cases where the High Court recognised that the employer's duty of care covered mental health as well as physical health is shown in *Box 20.1*. This case has been followed by further reports of payments for compensation for stress across a wide range of employment.

For example, in August 2000, it was reported that a bank manager was paid £100000 in an out-of-court settlement by Lloyds TSB after suffering intolerable stress at work (*The Times* 2000). In March 2003 (Ford 2003) an award of £150000 was agreed to be paid to a retired prison officer who claimed that he had suffered psychological trauma when dealing with sex offenders. He stated that he had not been properly supervised or prepared for this work. In another case involving the prison service, a prison clerk who saw a colleague held hostage by what she thought was an armed gang, without knowing they were prison officers on a training exercise, was awarded £100000 for stress. (*The Times* 2003)

Box 20.1. Stress at work:
Walker v. Northumberland County Council

A social worker obtained compensation when his employer failed to provide the necessary support in a stressful work situation when he returned to work following an earlier absence due to stress. The employer was not liable for the initial absence, but that put the employer on notice that the employee was vulnerable and its failure to provide the assistance he needed was a breach of its duty to provide reasonable care for his health and safety, as required under the contract of employment.

Court of Appeal rulings

Recent decisions of the Court of Appeal (*Hatton v. Sutherland and other cases* 2002) have clarified the law relating to compensation for stress at work. Four appeals were heard together by the Court of Appeal. In each one the employer appealed against a finding of liability for an employee's psychiatric illness caused by stress at work. Two of the claimants were teachers in public sector comprehensive schools, the third an administrative assistant at a local authority training centre and the fourth a raw material operative in a factory.

In determining whether the employer was liable or not, the Court of Appeal held that the ordinary principles of employer's liability applied to an allegation of psychiatric illness caused by stress at work. The threshold question was whether the particular kind of harm — an injury to health (as distinct to occupational health) which was attributable to stress at work (as distinct from other factors) — to the employee was reasonably foreseeable. Foreseeability depended upon what the employer knew or ought reasonably to have known about the individual employee. Because of the nature of mental disorder, it was harder to foresee than physical injury, but might be easier to foresee in a known individual than in the population at large. An employer was usually entitled to assume that the employee could withstand the normal pressures of his job unless he knew of some particular problem or vulnerability. The test was the same whatever the employment: there were no occupations which should be regarded as intrinsically dangerous to mental health.

The relevant factors identified by the Court of Appeal in determining the reasonable foreseeability of stress were:

- The nature and extent of the work done by the employee.
- The signs from the employee of impending harm to his health.

The employer was entitled to take at face value what he was told by an employee; he did not have to make searching inquiries of the employee or seek to make further inquiries of the employee's medical advisors.

If there were indications of impending harm to health arising from stress at work and these indications were plain enough for any reasonable employer to realise that he should do something about it, then the duty of the employer to take steps would be triggered. The employer could only be in breach of duty if he failed to take the steps which were reasonable in the circumstances, bearing in mind the magnitude of the risk of harm occurring, the gravity of the harm which might occur, the costs and practicability of preventing it and the justifications for running the risk. The factors to be taken into account in determining what was reasonable action by the employer included:

- The size and scope of the employer's operation, its resources, and the demands it faced.
- The interests of other employees.
- The need to treat other employees fairly (e.g. in any redistribution of duties).

An employer could reasonably be expected to take steps which were likely to do some good, and the court was likely to need expert evidence on that.

An employer who offered a confidential advice service, with referral to appropriate counselling or treatment services, was unlikely to be found in breach of duty. If the only reasonable and effective step would have been to dismiss or demote the employee, the employer would not be in breach of duty in allowing a willing employee to continue in the job.

In all cases it was necessary to identify the steps which the employer both could and should have taken before finding him in breach of his duty of care. The claimant had to show that the breach of duty had caused or materially contributed to the harm suffered. It was not enough to show that the occupational stress had caused the harm. Where the harm suffered had more than one cause, the employer should only pay for that proportion of the harm suffered which was attributable to his wrongdoing, unless the harm was truly indivisible. It was for the defendant to raise the question of apportionment. The assessment of damages would take account of any pre-existing disorder or vulnerability and of the chance that the claimant would have succumbed to a stress-related disorder in any event.

On the actual facts of the appeals before it, the Court of Appeal allowed the appeals by the employers in three cases and dismissed the appeal in the case of *Jones v. Sandwell Metropolitan Borough Council*. (In *Barber v. Somerset County Council,* Barber subsequently won his appeal in the House of Lords, see below.)

Comment on Court of Appeal decision

It could be seen as though the Court of Appeal has tightened the law relating to compensation for stress. A letter to *The Times* from the Chief Executive of the Mental After Care Association (Hitchon 2002) deplored the consequences of the decision 'because of the real danger that employers will use these rulings as an excuse to sit back and relax'. In fact, the Court has merely emphasised the basic law which has always applied to the duty of the employer to take reasonable care of the employee's health and safety. Because the duty is not an absolute one, but a reasonably practicable one, it is essential for the employee claiming compensation to be able to show that:

- The employer was aware of the situation the employee was in.
- It was reasonably foreseeable to the employer that serious mental harm to that particular employee could result.
- There was reasonable action which the employer could take to prevent the harm arising.
- The employer failed to take that action.
- The employer's failure to take that action caused the employee to suffer significant harm.

From the employer's perspective, it is essential that there should be comprehensive records of the action taken by the employer when it was made aware of the situation of the employee.

House of Lords decision: The Barber case

One of the employees whose case was lost in the Court of Appeal when the court upheld his employer's appeal succeeded in the House of Lords (*Barber v. Somerset County Council* 2004).

Mr Barber, the head of the Maths Department at East Bridgwater Community School, was involved in a restructuring of staffing at the school following which he became 'mathematical area of experience co-ordinator' and to maintain his salary level he had also taken on the post of project manager for public and media relations. To discharge all his responsibilities he was working between 61 and 70 hours a week. Stress took its toll and in the summer term of 1996 he was off sick for three weeks with sick notes showing 'overstressed/depression' and 'stress'. On his return to work he had filled in the council's form of sickness declaration stating his troubles as 'overstressed/depression'. He initiated a meeting with the headmistress, but found that she treated him unsympathetically by telling him that all the staff were under stress. Similarly, meetings with the two deputy heads, although more sympathetic, resulted in no steps being taken to improve or consider the situation beyond urging him to prioritise his work. In the autumn he found himself with the same or even possibly a slightly heavier workload. In November he lost control of himself and found himself shaking a pupil. He left school that day and never returned. Since then he has been unable to work as a teacher or do any work other than undemanding part-time work. He took early retirement in March 1997, aged 52 years.

The House of Lords held that the guidance issued by the Court of Appeal that unless the employer knows of some particular problem or vulnerability, he is usually entitled to assume that his employee is up to the normal pressures of the job, was only guidance and not a rule of law. Every case had to be decided on its own facts. The House of Lords quoted the principle established in an earlier case (*Stokes v. Guest* 1968):

The overall test is still the conduct of the reasonable and prudent employer taking positive thought for the safety of his workers in the light of what he knows or ought to know.

The House of Lords held (in a majority decision) that on the facts there had not been a flagrant breach of duty by the employer, but nor was it an obviously hopeless claim. It decided that there was insufficient reason for the Court of Appeal to set aside the decision of the High Court. At the very least, the school's senior management team should have taken the initiative in making sympathetic inquiries about him when he returned to work in June 1996, and make some reduction to his workload to ease his return. Even a small reduction in workload, coupled with the feeling that the team was on his side, might have made a difference. In any event, his condition should have been monitored and if it did not improve some more drastic action should have been taken.

A more recent Court of Appeal decision (*Young v. Post Office* 2002) dismissed an employer's appeal against a finding that it had breached its duty of care to the employee. The Court of Appeal held that the judge had been right to find that the Post Office owed a duty of care to Young, given its knowledge that Young's psychiatric problems were work related. The Post Office's failure to implement fully the agreed measures for Young's return to work were sufficiently serious to amount to a breach of that duty. Young was known to the Post Office to be both vulnerable and conscientious, which meant that he was likely to try to carry out his work without complaint, which meant that extra care should have been taken of him. No finding of contributory negligence was therefore appropriate.

In another case the Court of Appeal allowed the appeal of employers against a finding of liability for stress and an award of £30 856 (*Bonser v. UK Coal Mining Ltd*). The court held that for an employee to recover damages for psychiatric injury caused by stress at work, it had to be demonstrated that the employee had exhibited sufficient signs for it to be reasonably foreseeable by the employer that injury to health would result from the stress caused. The fact that in this case the employee was on an occasion tearful and upset did not make it reasonably foreseeable to the employer that stress would cause her to crack, as the trial judge had considered.

The Court of Appeal also allowed an appeal by a police constable who was required to attach a tagging device to a criminal's car while the criminal was in a pub and suffered a stroke precipitated by the stress of constantly having to change faulty batteries in the tagging device (*Donachie v. Chief Constable of Greater Manchester Police* 2004).

The Barber case was followed by the Court of Appeal in the case of *Dickins v O2 Plc* [2008]. In the case the Court of Appeal dismissed the employer's appeal against a finding that it was liable for psychiatric injury negligently caused by excessive stress in the course of her employment as a regulatory finance manager. She was awarded £109 754 which took into account a 50 percent reduction on account of other factors which had contributed to her illness.

Stress and unfair dismissal

The Court of Appeal held that a teacher who had won compensation in an application for unfair dismissal was able to bring an action at common law for compensation for breach of the employer's duty to take reasonable care of his health which led him to suffer from a psychiatric disorder (*McCabe v. Cornwall CC* 2002). The Court of Appeal held that an employee was not automatically barred for bringing a common law action in respect of the employer's conduct leading up to the dismissal. Cornwall County Council's appeal was dismissed in the House of Lords. The House of Lords held that where an employer had acted unfairly towards an employee, in such a way that the employee had acquired a cause of action at common law prior to and independently of his subsequent unfair dismissal, his common law action was not barred by the existence of his statutory unfair dismissal claim (*Eastwood and another* 2004). This principle is important since the House of Lords has held that in an unfair dismissal claim, the statutory provisions of the Employment Rights Act 1996 mean the employee can only recover compensation for pecuniary loss (*Dunnachie v. Kingston upon Hull City Council* 2004) (see *Chapter 6*).

Grounds for obtaining compensation for stress

To establish grounds for compensation for stress induced by work on the basis of his/her common law rights, an employee would have to show:

- That he/she was under an unacceptable level of stress at work.
- That the employer was aware of this situation.
- That there was reasonable action which the employer could have taken to relieve this pressure.
- That the employer failed to take that action.
- That as a result the employee has suffered a serious mental condition.

In other words, like any other situation of health and safety in the workplace, the employee is entitled to rely upon the four elements in any negligence action which were considered in *Chapter 5*, i.e. duty owed by the employer to safeguard the health and safety of the employee, breach of the duty, causation and harm.

Following the inquest on a consultant who was exhausted from working up to 100 hours a week and who died after injecting himself with anaesthetic whilst on duty at hospital, the British Medical Association announced that it was stepping up its campaign to restrict doctors' hours (Wright 2003a).

Bennett et al (1999) provide advice on handling stress. They emphasise the importance of looking at the work environment and personal skills as part of any stress management strategy.

Counselling services

The House of Lords made it clear in the Hatton case that the offering of counselling services by the employer was not in itself sufficient action to ensure that there was no breach of duty by the employer. In the case of *Daw v. Intel Corporation* [2007], the Court of Appeal observed that the reference to counselling services in Hatton did not make such services a panacea by which employers can discharge their duty of care in all cases. In that case, the judge had been entitled to hold the employer in breach notwithstanding that it provided a counselling service. The employee's problems could only be dealt with by management intervention.

In the case of *Paterson v. Surrey Police Authority* [2008] the High Court judge could find no causal element between any breach of duty by the police employers and the breakdown of Mr Paterson and he therefore failed in his claim. The police authority had no duty to offer him alternative accommodation which was the cause of his psychiatric illness.

Health and safety prosecutions and stress

In August 2003, the Health and Safety Executive issued its first enforcement notice against an NHS hospital for failing to protect doctors and nurses from stress at work (de Bruxelles et al 2003). Dorset Hospitals NHS Trust was given until 15 December 2003 to assess stress levels among its 1100 staff and introduce a programme to reduce it. If it failed to act it would face court action and fines under the Health and Safety at Work Act 1974.

The HSE in 2002 published a report which provided examples of how sources of work stress were identified and managed in a number of hospital settings. The report provides an account of the risk management process using these case study examples. It shows how risk management can be a powerful tool for dealing with sources of work stress.

In June 2003 the Health and Safety Executive published draft management standards (risk assessment tool) which suggested methods by which employers could reduce stress in the workplace. The standards were piloted in 2003. The HSE defines them in the following terms:

The Management Standards define the characteristics, or culture, of an organisation where the risks from work-related stress are being effectively managed and controlled.

During the piloting of the Management Standards the HSE launched Real Solutions, Real People which is a manager's guide to tackling work-related stress, based around a series of case studies and which can be downloaded from the website (www.hse.gov.uk/stress/issues.htm). The guide for employers in making the management standards work was published in October 2010. The six management standards cover: demands, control, support, role, change and relationships. An HSE guide for employees first published in 2005 and updated in 2008 *Working Together at Work to Reduce Stress* explains the management standards from an employee perspective, outlines the role of the employee in stress management and the action an employee should take if he or she feels stressed.

The steps which the HSE recommend should be taken are as follows:

- Step 1: Identify the risk factors.
- Step 2: Who can be harmed and how?
- Step 3: Evaluate the risks.
- Step 4: Record your findings.
- Step 5: Monitor and review.

Guidance provided by the HSE and available on its website includes case studies of how various organisations have developed strategies of reducing work-related stress. These include examples of health service organisations including the Great Western Hospitals NHS Foundation Trust (formerly Swindon and Marlborough NHS Trust) and Harrogate and District NHS Foundation Trust.

Surveys were carried out by the Commission for Healthcare Audit of Inspection, now the Care Quality Commission (CQC), as part of their inspections to monitor stress levels. The CQC was responsible for setting up the 7th annual survey of NHS staff and stated:

> This is the seventh annual survey of NHS staff. It provides trusts with information about the views and experiences of employees that can help to improve the working lives of staff and the quality of care for patients. Almost 290000 NHS staff were asked for their views on working in the NHS in October 2009 (55 percent responded). The Care Quality Commission will use the results from the survey in a range of ways including: setting out national findings informing patients and the public of trusts' results using the results in regulatory activities such as registration, the monitoring of ongoing compliance, and reviews. The Department of Health will also use the results to inform commissioning, service improvement and performance measurement, and to review and inform NHS policies.

The CQC reported on the results of the 7th survey noting that:

We also see a small increase in staff job satisfaction and a decrease in the proportion of staff who say they are thinking of leaving their trust. There has been a fall in, for example, the proportion of staff: feeling pressure at work (a small drop in the scale score); working extra hours (down by one percentage point); experiencing physical violence from patients/relatives in last the 12 months (down by one percentage point); experiencing harassment, bullying or abuse from patients/relatives in last the 12 months (down by one percentage point). The experience of staff has deteriorated in two key findings with a one percentage point drop in the proportion of staff receiving job-relevant training, learning or development in the previous 12 months and in the proportion of staff feeling able to contribute towards improvements at work.

It is clear that CQC will continue to monitor stress levels within the NHS which are part of its quality monitoring.

The HSE estimated that British industry loses £370 million a year because of stress, while the cost to society as a whole could be £3.75 billion (Wright 2003b).

Application of the law to *Scenario 20.1*

With reference to *Scenario 20.1*, it should not be concluded that after a few nights of insomnia Iris could obtain compensation for stress from her employer. Iris would have to show that she was suffering from a significant mental illness as a result of stress at work, that her employers were aware of the situation and that there was reasonable action which her managers could have taken but failed to take. She does not have to wait until she becomes seriously ill before taking action. She should make it known to her managers that she is in an impossible situation. It would then be the manager's responsibility to assess the situation and to decide on the reasonable action which could be taken to relieve the pressure upon Iris and her colleagues. It may be that there would have to be discussions with the trust board over reducing the number of intensive care beds. If no reasonable action is taken to protect and support Iris, she may be able to argue that the employers are in fundamental breach of their contractual duties towards her and that this gives her the right to see herself as constructively dismissed, which would enable her to go to an employment tribunal for unfair dismissal.

Bullying

Scenario 20.2. Stress at work

Poppy had just completed her midwiery training and had started work as a staff midwife in Roger Park Hospital. She found that one of the senior midwives was inclined to bully her, ordering her around, failing to give her clear instructions and then blaming her if things were not done. When she talked to other staff, they simply shrugged and said that that was what she was like and she should get used to the situation. Poppy is finding that the situation is becoming impossible, that she is losing what little confidence she had as a newly qualified midwife and feels that her only option is to change jobs, even though her present post is ideally suited to her personal circumstances. What can she do legally?

Employers' duty to prevent bullying

The duty owed by the employer to the employee to take reasonable care of the health and safety of the employee also includes the duty to protect the employee against bullying. There have recently been several payments of compensation in respect of employers' failures to take action to control bullying. For example, in one case, £100000 was accepted in an out-of-court settlement by a teacher who alleged that he had been bullied by the headteacher and other staff, when he was teaching in a school in Pembrokeshire (*The Times* 1998). Another teacher who was bullied by her headmistress was awarded £86,000 (Halpin 2003).

Bullying may be associated with racial or other harassment. In November 2001, it was reported that two senior midwives in Portsmouth were dismissed following allegations of harassment and bullying (Practising Midwife 2001). Preliminary findings of research carried out by Professor Mavis Kirkham of Sheffield University's Informed Childbearing and Health Research Group, commissioned by the Royal College of Midwives, into why midwives leave the NHS has shown evidence of bullying by senior midwives. The Andrea Adams Trust, a support organisation which helps health service employees, has provided a fact sheet on workplace bullying (Andrea Adams Trust 2000). An overview of workplace bullying in midwifery departments and how it may be addressed is provided by Ruth Hadikin (Hadikin 2001). She provides an action checklist for targets of workplace bullying. Records are, of course, essential. From the results of a survey published in the British Medical Journal (Quine 1999), it was concluded that bullying in a community NHS trust was a serious problem and setting up systems for supporting staff and for dealing with interpersonal conflict may have benefits for both employees and staff. (The Andrea Adams Trust has since ceased to operate as a charity and its suggests that persons seeking help should contact ACAS.)

Responsibilities of employers and managers

Employers should ensure that there is an organisation-wide policy on preventing and eradicating bullying. Managers, as representatives of the employer, have a responsibility to be sensitive to situations of both stress and bullying. They must ensure that they take control of the situation and all reasonable action is taken to support the afflicted employee. In certain circumstances the manager may need to use disciplinary action to warn an employee who is bullying others. The disciplinary procedure must be followed and advice taken from human resources over how it should be applied. It may be that counselling is appropriate initially, but if this is ineffective, the manager might have to give an oral warning or first written warning to the employee. If such action is ineffective, eventually there may be grounds for dismissing the bully. If the bully were to claim that the dismissal was unfair, then evidence of the disciplinary action taken, and the justification for it, would be essential before the employment tribunal to provide evidence of both the reason for the dismissal and also the reasonableness of the employer's action in treating that reason as justifying dismissal. Inevitably, the documentation identifying exactly what occurred and the action which was taken is extremely important as evidence if there are legal proceedings. In certain severe situations it may be necessary to carry out a major internal or external investigation as to what is happening within a unit. For example, an investigation was instigated into allegations of bullying in a cardiac unit at Morriston Hospital, Swansea. Fifteen operations were rescheduled after the unit closed to all but emergency cases (Barkham 2004). The HSE has provided guidance for individuals and employers on bullying which may often be linked with work-related stress and is available on its dedicated website for stress (www.hse.gov.uk/stress). The HSE describes the impact of bullying:

> *It can result in psychological health problems such as depression, anxiety or low self-esteem It can result in physical health problems such as stomach problems,*

or sleep difficulties If you've witnessed the bullying of a colleague, this can also be very upsetting and can impact on your health. Your performance at work can be affected.

The HSE outlines the action which an employee can take, including discussing the situation with someone within the organisation that he or she feels comfortable with, and trying to resolve the situation informally or by mediation and if this fails by taking legal action. However it warns of the complexity of legal action. It advises of other resources for advice and assistance including ACAS.

Application of the law to *Scenario 20.2*

In *Scenario 20.2*, Poppy is entitled to have the support of her manager in dealing with the situation which she finds intolerable and stressful. All that has been said above in relation to Iris applies to Poppy's legal position. Poppy needs to document exactly how she is being bullied and the effects that it is having upon her and give the full details to her manager. The latter may well attempt to deal with the bully by an initial counselling session with the assistance of the personnel department. There may be training sessions on personal management and communications which the bully could be advised to attend. Poppy could be given positive help in terms of developing her assertion and coping skills. If the situation does not improve, the next stage would be disciplinary action against the bully. Ultimately, the final sanction would be dismissal, which may be challenged in an employment tribunal. The documentation of all that has taken place would be vital evidence.

Conclusions

The duty placed upon the employer to take reasonable action to protect the employee's mental as well as physical health is clearly established by the successful claims for compensation for stress and bullying. A new development, however, is the action taken by the Health and Safety Executive to issue notices where NHS organisations are failing to carry out risk assessments on stress. This initiative may well lead to greater concentration by employers on a growing concern.

The disastrous effects of work-related stress and workplace bullying are well recognised by the courts and by health and safety, employer and employee organisations and health professional associations. However there is evidence that the stress and bullying are endemic in the NHS and more vigorous and sustained action needs to be taken to control and eliminate it. The Protection from Harassment Act 1997 may also be of value to victims and it is to this we look in the next chapter on violence.

References

Andrea Adams Trust (2000) *Factsheet on workplace bullying*. Andrea Adams Trust (The Charity has since closed down)

Barber v. Somerset County Council 2004. The Times Law Report 5 April 2004 HL

Barkham P (2004) Bullying inquiry at closed NHS unit. *The Times* 5 March

Bennett P, Scott L, Harling K (1999) Stress busters. *Nursing Times* 95(50): 28–9

Bonser v. UK Coal Mining Ltd (Formerly RJB Mining (UK) Ltd) The Times Law Report 30 June 2003 CA

Daw v. Intel Corporation [2007] ICR 1318

de Bruxelles S, Wright O, Rumbelow H (2003) Bosses will be fined for workers' stress. *The Times*, 5 August

Dickins v O2 Plc [2008] EWCA Civ 1144

Donachie v. Chief Constable of Greater Manchester Police 2004 The Times Law Report 6 May 2004

Dunnachie v. Kingston upon Hull City Council 2004 The Times Law Report 16 July 2004

Eastwood and Another v. Magnox Electric plc, McCabe v. Cornwall County Council and Another 2004. The Times Law Report 16 July 2004

Ford R (2003) Prison Officer wins £150,000 trauma payout. *The Times* 1 April

Hadikin R (2001) MIDIRS (The Midwives Information and Resource Service). *Midwifery Digest* 11(3): 308–11

Halpin T (2003) Teacher bullied by head awarded £86,000. *The Times*, 18 November

Hatton v. Sutherland, Barber v. Somerset County Council, Jones v. Sandwell Metropolitan Borough Council, Baker v. Baker Refractories Ltd (2002) The Times Law Report 12 February; [2002] EWCA 76 [2002] 2 All ER 1

Health and Safety Executive (2002) CRR 435/2002 *Interventions to Control Stress at Work in Hospital Staff*. HSE, London

Health and Safety Executive (2003) *Real Solutions, Real People – A manager's guide to tackling work-related stress*. HSE, London

Hitchon G (2002) Letter to the editor. *The Times* 19 February

McCabe v. Cornwall CC [2002] EWCA Civ 1887; The Times 28 December 2002 CA

Paterson v. Surrey Police Authority [2008] EWHC 2693 (QB)

Practising Midwife (2001) News item. *Practising Midwife* 4(10): 6

Quine L (1999) Workplace bullying in NHS community trust: Staff questionnaire survey. *British Medical Journal* 318: 228–32

Stokes v. Guest, Keen and Nettlefold (Bolts and Nuts) Ltd [1968] 1 WLR 1776,

Sutherland V, Cooper CL (2003) *Practical Stress Management for Doctors*. Butterworth Heinemann, London

The Times (1998) Victoria Fletcher teacher 'bullied by staff' wins £100,000. News report. *The Times* 17 July

The Times (2000) Elizabeth Judge Banker wins £100,000 stress payout. *The Times* 10 August

The Times (2003) News Item. Jail clerk's £100,000 for stress. *The Times*

Walker v. Northumberland County Council (1994) The Times Law Report 24 November, Queen's Bench Division; [1995] 1 All ER 737

Wright O (2003a) Doctor worn out by 'crazy hours' took fatal overdose. *The Times* 17 May 2003

Wright O (2003b) CBI backs employers over new stress law. *The Times* 6 August 2003

Young v. Post Office (2002) EWCA Civ 661 (2002) IRLR 660

CHAPTER 21

Violence

Scenario 21.1. Violence in A&E

May, a doctor in the accident and emergency department, was on duty at the weekend when a patient was brought in by two friends. It was clear that they had all been drinking heavily. It appeared that the patient had serious injuries following a fall. May attempted to arrange for the patient to be taken into a cubicle, but in so doing was struck by one of the friends and suffered a serious blow to her face. What rights does she have in law?

Introduction

The level of reported violence against health service staff both in hospital and in the community has been increasing over recent years. There are approximately 65 000 incidents against NHS staff each year, 64 percent against nursing staff (Department of Health 2001). This prompted Alan Milburn, the Secretary of State for Health, to announce in a press release in December 2001 that it was justifiable for health staff to refuse to treat patients who were violent, drunk and abusive to them (Department of Health 2001). The NHS Security and Management Service (NHS SMS) (see below) publishes annual figures. Those for 2009/10 show that there were 56 718 assaults on staff with the ratio per 1000 staff ranging from 14 per 1000 staff in primary care trusts to 16.8 in acute care and 191.7 in mental health care.

The Government has launched a zero tolerance zone campaign (see more details below) to tackle violence in the NHS. National Guidelines on withholding treatment from violent and abusive patients in NHS trusts have been issued by the Department of Health (obtainable from the zero tolerance website). The rules relating to the terms of service of GPs have been changed to enable them to arrange for the removal from their list of any patient who threatens violence to them. In 2003 the National Audit Office reported that reports of violence against NHS staff have risen by 13 percent in two years, costing the service at least £69 million annually (National Audit Office 2003). The report estimated that about 40 percent of incidents were not being reported. The British Medical Association reported in October 2003 that one in 10 doctors is assaulted every year (British Medical Association 2003). Those most likely to be assaulted were those working in A&E departments, in psychiatric services and in general practice.

Some of the examples of death or serious injury include:

- The case where a voluntary patient at a mental hospital was charged with assault occasioning actual bodily harm to an occupational therapist employed at the hospital (*R v. Lincolnshire (Kesteven) Justices, ex parte Connor* [1983]).
- A case where an occupational therapist was killed by a mentally ill patient in the Edith Morgan Unit at Torbay; an inquiry was set up following this death (Blom-Cooper et al 1995).
- A case where a health care assistant was attacked in the grounds of a Bristol hospital (Mahoney 2000). Her assailant was jailed for 10 years (*The Times* 2001).

Duty of the employer

The employer has a duty to take reasonable care of employees in relation to reasonably foreseeable violence. A risk assessment would therefore be required of this possibility and as a result any reasonable means to protect the employee should be adopted.

Guidance prepared by the Health and Safety Commission gave practical advice for reducing the risk of violence in a variety of settings, and emphasises the importance of commitment from highest levels of management (Health and Safety Commission 1997). In 2010 the HSE published a report by Packham. It did so

> ...as part of its responsibility for developing and implementing policy on work-related violence. The HSE has published a wide range of guidance on the prevention and management of work-related violence, and works in partnership with others (including the Home Office, other Government departments, employers, trades unions and local authorities), to raise awareness of the issue and share good practice.

The figures from the British Crime Survey showed that whilst the overall level of violence was 1.4 percent of working adults in the year 2009/10, police had a much higher level of 9.0 percent, health professionals 3.8 percent, and health and social welfare associate professionals 2.6 percent. Strangers were the offenders in 65 percent of cases of workplace violence and, according to the victims, 38 percent of the attackers were under the influence of alcohol and 19 percent under the influence of drugs.

In October 1998, it was reported that North West Durham Health Care Trust was to meet the full legal costs and provide emotional and professional support for all health care staff who take court action against an assailant in cases where the Crown Prosecution Service (CPS) fails to pursue the offender (Frean 1998). However, there would appear to be good grounds for any such prosecution to be undertaken by the CPS. This would spare an individual employee the cost and risk of the prosecution.

In October 2000, the Department of Health announced guidelines to tackle violence against NHS staff who are most at risk. The guidelines covered:

- Risk assessment.
- Crime prevention.
- Protection of NHS staff in the community.
- Techniques for dealing with abusive and potentially violent situations.
- Training.
- Reporting of incidents.
- The criminal justice system.
- Support for victims.

New guidance has been issued by the NHS Security Management Service (see below)

Protection of staff

The employer's duty is to provide all reasonable care of the employee from reasonably foreseeable violence or abuse. What is reasonable depends upon the actual circumstances of the reasonably foreseeable violence. There are examples of what some employers have provided: ambulance staff in London are being issued with anti-stab vests for occasions when they enter addresses on a high risk list (Studd 2003). The vests are being issued (at a cost of £1 million) as part of a wider campaign to protect ambulance staff from the 400 assaults they suffer each year. The police were investigating the possibility of introducing leg restraints to see if they can reduce injuries from violent prisoners after arrests. Sussex police were testing a system that used velcro straps and another known as the Viper (Violent Persons Restraint System) which uses webbing to hold the arms and ankles (Tendler 1999).

Protection from Harassment Act 1997

This Act creates certain offences and civil wrongs which are shown in *Box 21.1*.

Certain defences are permitted in the Act, including if an individual is preventing or detecting crime. The court has held that a company could not be the victim of harassment, only an individual (*Dalichi UK Ltd and others v. Stop Huntingdon Animal Cruelty and Other*s 2003).

Duties and training of staff

Every employee has a responsibility to ensure that any concerns about aggression and violence are brought to the attention of the management and that action is taken. In certain circumstances it may be that there should be training for

---

Box 21.1: Protection from Harassment Act 1997

1 A criminal offence of harassment (Section 1), which is defined as a person pursuing a course of conduct that amounts to harassment of another and that he knows or ought to know amounts to harassment of the other (the reasonable person test is applied);

2 A civil wrong whereby a person who fears an actual or future breach of Section 1, may claim compensation including damages for anxiety and financial loss;

3 The right to claim an injunction to restrain the defendant from pursuing any conduct that amounts to harassment;

4 The right to apply for a warrant for the arrest of the defendant, if the injunction has not been obeyed;

5 It creates an offence of putting people in fear of violence, where a person causes by his conduct another person to fear on at least two occasions that violence will be used against him;

6 Restraining orders can be made by the court for the purpose of protecting the victim of the offence or any other person from further conduct amounting to harassment or to fear of violence.

---

employees to defuse a potentially violent situation. For example, Steve McHale, an aggression management co-ordinator, emphasised that nurses themselves must develop the skills to defuse rather than build up aggression (McHale 1999). He stated that:

> *The main causes of aggression against nurses are the patient's loss of control or autonomy over a situation, a feeling of depersonalisation and a lack of communication.*

Schools have enlisted staff from high-security hospitals to train teachers to deal with disruptive children as young as five years old (O'Leary 1999).

In the community, health professionals would have a duty to warn colleagues of potential dangers and they might therefore record in their notes that it may be advisable for a second person to accompany the health professional for the next house call. The duty of confidentiality owed to the patient would be subject to an exception in the public interest where a health professional needed to warn colleagues about a fear of violence from a particular patient. The London ambulance service was the first in the country to introduce self-defence training (Studd 2003).

Rights of the employee

The employer's duty extends to protecting the employee against reasonably foreseeable attacks from violent patients or even from violent visitors and violent trespassers. It is not an absolute duty, but a reasonably practicable one. To obtain compensation from an NHS trust the employee must establish that either the NHS trust was itself directly at fault in failing to take reasonable action to protect him/her from violence, or that another employee has been negligent in the course of employment and therefore the NHS trust is vicariously liable. The health professional would need to provide evidence that:

- There were reasonable precautions that the authority could have taken and failed to take, e.g. male staffing on mixed wards, training in the handling of violent patients, improved security services support; or
- Special facilities for dealing with known aggressive patients should have been provided, e.g. a special wing, an alarm system, a safe system for control of dangerous items; or
- Inadequate staffing was provided in areas where violence could be

reasonably foreseen, e.g. in dangerous estates in the community, in psychiatric wards, in accident and emergency departments.

In addition to showing the absence of reasonable measures to protect them, injured employees would also have to show that there was a causal connection between the injuries suffered and these failures on the authority's part. In other words, they would have to show that had these precautions been taken, they would probably not have suffered any injury. In its defence, the NHS trust would have to establish either that such reasonable precautions had been provided – a dispute on the facts – or that even if such precautions had been taken the injury would still have occurred. In addition, it might be able to show that the health professional was contributorily negligent (*Chapter 5*).

Suing the aggressor

Could the health professional sue the aggressor if he/she has been injured by an assault?

The answer is that the health professional would have a right of action against anyone who assaults him/her, but there are difficulties where the aggressor is a patient who is mentally disordered. The Magistrates Courts have thrown out such cases as being inappropriate. If the defendant is prosecuted, the magistrate or judge can make an order for compensation to be paid by the defendant to the injured person. Any civil action for compensation, however, is not recommended if the defendant does not have the resources to pay.

In addition, the health professional injured as a result of a criminal act has the right to seek compensation from the Criminal Injuries Compensation Authority. This body pays out compensation according to a tariff of payments (see *Chapter 7*).

Self-defence

Can the health professional defend him/herself if attacked by a patient, visitor, trespasser or employee?

Every citizen has the right of self-defence. The health professional could use reasonable means to defend him/herself against an aggressor. Reasonableness means, first, that the force used should be no more than is necessary to accomplish the object for which it is allowed (so retaliation, revenge and punishment are not permitted) and, second, the reaction must be in proportion to the harm which is threatened. Thus, all the circumstances must be taken into account: the contrast between the strength, size, expertise of the assailant and the defendant; and the type of harm with which the person is being threatened.

Obviously, the greater the severity of the threatened danger, the more reasonable it is to take tougher measures. In assessing the reasonableness of the defence, account is taken of the fact that the defendant may only have a brief period to make up his/her mind what to do.

Zero tolerance zone

The Department of Health has set up a dedicated website (www.dh.gov.uk/ zerotolerance/) to provide information and support for health service bodies to wipe out threats and violence to NHS staff. The website provides resources and guidance for managers and staff in developing and implementing a local zero tolerance policy. The website has two specific aims:

* To get over to the public that violence against staff working in the NHS is unacceptable and the Government is determined to stamp it out; and
* To get over to all staff that violence and intimidation is unacceptable and is being tackled.

The zero tolerance site provides a list of issues which should be included in any local policy. These include:

* A pledge to protect staff at work.
* The definition of violence.
* Details of the employers' legal requirements.
* Details of managers' and employees' responsibilities.
* Information on risk assessment measures.
* Details of local prevention and reduction plans and local emergency procedures.
* An explanation of staff training and local reporting procedures.

Examples are given of successful prosecutions brought against individuals assaulting NHS staff. Funds have been allocated by the Department of Health to assist staff in bringing private prosecutions, if there are no public prosecutions (Lister 2003). The Public Accounts Committee has recommended that victims of assault should be offered counselling and be supported to take perpetrators to court (Public Accounts Committee 2003). The Royal College of Nursing issued on 27 March 2003 a press release in response to the National Audit Office report, *Safer Place to Work,* emphasising the RCN's commitment to protecting nursing staff from violence and calling upon improved support from managers and a consistent approach to the problem (www.rcn.org.uk/news/media).

Refusing treatment

Ultimately, health professionals have the power to refuse a violent patient treatment. The guidelines set out in the zero tolerance site should be followed. GPs can require a patient who is aggressive and violent to be removed from the GP list. In June 2004, the Court ordered the banning of a man from every hospital and doctor's surgery in England and Wales (Lister 2004). Norman Hutchins was prohibited from entering or making contact with any NHS or private medical centre. He was also barred from seeking medical clothing or equipment. He had been accused of upsetting staff on 47 occasions since November 2003 in his endeavours to obtain medical clothing and equipment. He was placed initially on a four-week interim anti-social behaviour order pending a full hearing at the end of June 2004 (Norfolk 2004). The order was sought by the NHS Counter Fraud and Security Management Service which was established in 2003 and set up a new system for reporting physical and verbal attacks in November 2003.

NHS Counter Fraud and Security Management Service and the NHS Security Management Service

The Security Management Service (SMS) is part of the Counter Fraud and Security Management Service (CFSMS), which is an independent division of the NHS Business Services Authority. The NHS SMS was originally launched in April 2003 with a remit encompassing all policy and operational responsibility for the management of security in the NHS (Statutory Instrument 3039/2002). It describes its remit as broad and defines it as

> protecting people and property, so that the highest standards of clinical care can be made available to patients.

Before April 2003, security management work fell to various parts of the Department of Health and the NHS, or was not addressed at all. For the first time, security management has been brought under the direction of one central organisation within the NHS. In March 2004 the Commission for Health

Improvement (since April 2009 CQC) (www.cqc.gov.uk) published figures indicating that 15 percent of NHS staff reported experiencing violence at work during the previous year. In the light of these figures, the NHS Security Management Service (NHS SMS) published a new strategy which set out violence against NHS staff as the top priority to be tackled. From 2004 the NHS SMS has begun a vast training programme for NHS staff on conflict resolution, providing them with the skills to defuse potentially violent situations and training local security management specialists to deal with violence locally. It has also published some useful documents giving advice on managing and preventing violence. These include:

* *Tackling Violence Against Staff. Explanatory notes for reporting procedures introduced by the Secretary of State's Directions 'Protecting your NHS'* (first published 2003 and updated 2009).
* A Consultation Paper on marking the electronic care records of violent patients.
* *Not Alone – A guide for the better protection for lone workers in the NHS* (Revised 2009).

In February 2011 the Department of Health announced that it had commissioned the Design Centre to look at the design of A&E Departments with a view to developing innovative new ways to reduce violence and aggression towards NHS staff. The project will involve designers, architects, health care experts, patients and frontline NHS staff working together to develop and trial potential solutions.

Application of the law to *Scenario 21.1*

In *Scenario 21.1*, May has been injured as a result of violence by a visitor to the hospital. The various measures available to her are set out in *Box 21.2*. There is no reason why all of them should not be pursued. If, however, she obtains compensation from the criminal injuries compensation authority, this would take into account compensation which she receives through alternative claims.

Conclusion

It is disappointing that in spite of a zero tolerance campaign to eradicate violence from the health services, there is no sign that the number of injuries suffered by health services staff is reducing. Concerted efforts nationally and locally are still required to make it clear to the public that staff cannot be treated as punch

---

Box 21.2. Remedies for an employee following a violent incident

- Obtain compensation from the criminal courts following a successful prosecution of the assailant
- Sue the aggressor personally for trespass to the person (there is little point if he/she has no assets or income to pay the damages awarded)
- Seek compensation from the employer if it can be established that there has been a breach of the employer's duty to take reasonable care of her health and safety and protect her from violence
- Claim compensation from the Criminal Injuries Compensation Authority (see *Chapter 7*)
- Obtain statutory sick pay, sickness pay under NHS National agreements and Department of Social Security benefits for accidents at work

---

bags and that action will be taken against violence which is often associated with excess drinking. Health professionals should ensure that they are confident of their rights to have reasonable protection from such incidents. Clearly, evidence of what actually happened is essential to maintain a successful prosecution of the aggressor and support a health professional's claim for compensation. If a health professional is involved in violence or witnesses a violent incident, it is essential that a report and statement are completed and that the incident is fully documented.

References

Blom-Cooper L, Hally H, Murphy E (1995) *The Falling Shadow – One Patient's Mental Health Care*. Duckworth, London

British Medical Association (2003) V*iolence at Work: The experience of UK doctors*. BMA, London

Daiichi UK Ltd and others v. Stop Huntingdon Animal Cruelty and Others. Times Law Report 22 October 2003

Department of Health (2000) *Department of Health Guidance on Tackling Violence*. Department of Health, London (NHS Response Line 08701 555455)

Department of Health (2001) V*iolence Against NHS Staff 'Will Not be Tolerated'*. Press Release 2001/0644. 27 December 2001. Department of Health, London

Frean A (1998) Funds for nurses who prosecute violent patients. *The Times* 1 October

Health and Safety Commission (1997) *Violence and Aggression to Staff in Health*

Services. HSE Books, London

Lister S (2003) Ministers to fund action on abusive patients. *The Times* 15 April

Lister S (2004) Court to ban fetishist from health units. *The Times* 2 June

McHale S (1999) From insult to injury. *Nursing Times* 95(49): 30

Mahoney C (2000) Scene of HCA attack was secure. *Nursing Times* 96(6): 5

National Audit Office (2003) *A Safer Place to Work: protecting NHS Hospital and Ambulance Staff from Violence and Aggression*. Report of the Comptroller and Auditor General HC 527 Session 2002-2003 27 March 2003

Norfolk A (2004) Surgical mask fetishist banned from NHS. The Times 3 June

Packham C (2010) *Violence at Work: Findings from the 2009/10 British Crime Survey.* HSE Books, London

Public Accounts Committee (2003) A *Safer Place to Work: Improving the management of health and safety risks to staff in NHS Trusts*. Available from: www.publications. parliament.uk

O'Leary J (1999) Teachers to seek help with violent pupils. *The Times* 2 April

R v. Lincolnshire (Kesteven) Justices, ex parte Connor [1983] 1 All ER 901 QBD

Studd H (2003) Ambulance staff to get anti-stab vests. *The Times* 24 January

Tendler S (1999) Restraints tested to reduce injuries. *The Times* 2 April

The Times (2001) News Item. Ten years for nurse's attacker. *The Times* 2 June

CHAPTER 22

Smoking

> ### Scenario 22.1. The community health professional and the smoking patient
>
> A community nurse went to an elderly man's home every day to give him insulin injections and to attend to dressings for his leg ulcer. She complained that he smoked incessantly, that the house was filled with smoke and that after her visit her chest tightened up and she frequently suffered from an asthma attack. She wondered if she could refuse to visit this particular patient.

Introduction

Tobacco companies in the USA have been successfully sued by smokers who have claimed that as a result of the addiction and smoking-induced illnesses, they have suffered crippling and fatal illnesses. The millions of dollars awarded might well take some time for the litigants to receive because of the appeal process. The widow of a smoker lost her test case in 2005 against Imperial Tobacco. Alfred McTear who died of lung cancer in 1993 at the age of 48 had smoked 60 cigarettes a day. He had initiated the case before he died arguing that he was not aware of the link between smoking and lung cancer. His widow continued the case after his death (*McTear v. Imperial Tobacco Ltd* [2005]).

This chapter considers the law relating to smoking in the workplace, the rights of patients to be protected from passive smoking and, conversely, the rights of patients to smoke, and Government initiatives to assist people in giving up smoking.

Smoking in the workplace

The statutory duty of the employer under section 2 of the Health and Safety at Work Act 1974 states:

It shall be the duty of every employer to ensure, so far as is reasonably practicable, the health, safety and welfare at work of all his employees.

(See Chapter 2)

This statutory duty could be seen as requiring the employer to provide a smoke-free environment for employees to work in and this has been reinforced by legislation prohibiting smoking in public places (see below). A smoke-free environment is practicable in hospital premises, where smoking is forbidden, but may not be practicable in other environments. Bar staff are now entitled to work in a smoke-free environment since this right has been incorporated in law with the prohibition of smoking in public places (see below). The prohibition on smoking in public places has profound implications for smokers in pubs and restaurants. Failure by an employer to provide a smoke-free environment could lead to civil action for compensation by an employee. The employee (or the relatives of an employee who died as a result of passive smoking in the workplace) would have to prove that:

- Under the contract of employment, the employer had a duty to take reasonable care of the health and safety of the employee, and that this duty included providing a smoke-free environment.
- The employer was in breach of this contractual duty.
- As a consequence of this breach of duty, the employee had suffered reasonably foreseeable harm.
- The harm is significant personal injury or death.

The causation element would probably be the most difficult to establish; to prove that a particular disease or harm has been caused because of a smoke-filled atmosphere at work would require medical evidence that this was the main reason for the patient's ill-health.

Smoke-filled community premises

While a health professional is entitled to work in a smoke-free environment in hospital premises, the health professional who works in the community has a much more difficult task. *Scenario 22.1* is not an atypical situation for some community health professionals. Clearly, since these premises are not under the control of the employer of the community nurse, the employer does not have the right to insist that the patient gives up smoking, creating a smoke-free environment. Nor could it be said that a person's home is a public place. On the other hand, for the nurse it is her workplace and there is action that the employer can take to support the nurse. It might be possible to suggest that the patient should not smoke during the nurse's visit, and that he agrees to open windows and ventilate the room just before or when the nurse arrives. The employer may also be able to rearrange shifts, so that the duty of visiting this patient is shared with other community nurses who may be less sensitive to a smoking environment.

If such measures are taken, there should be no question of the community nurse refusing to visit this patient. This would be contrary to the NMC Code (Nursing and Midwifery Council 2008). If such measures were not taken, the community nurse should still not withdraw her services but should ask her manager to support her right to have reasonable care taken of her health and safety. If necessary, she may need to make use of the procedure set up under the Public Interest Disclosure Act 1998 to press her concerns (see *Chapter 23*).

Rights of patients to smoke

Not everyone supports a smoke-free environment and some patients, especially in psychiatric wards, who may be resident for several weeks, are not prepared or are unable to give up smoking during their admission. The author explored the right of a hospital to enforce a no-smoking policy on the premises and the dangers of not creating a smoking room in the context of antenatal services where pregnant women may be admitted for several weeks before the birth (Dimond 1996).

The conclusion was reached that while the occupier of the premises has the right (now the legal duty) to forbid smoking on the premises, to enforce this without providing a well-ventilated smoking area may be extremely dangerous. Patients who are desperate to smoke may, without well-ventilated segregated facilities for smoking, attempt to smoke in unauthorised places, such as treatment rooms and oxygen stores, thereby creating a hazardous situation. However the Court of Appeal decision has held that patients at the high security hospital Rampton did not have a human right to smoke and their appeal was dismissed. The patients had argued that the policy of prohibiting smoking in the premises of an NHS trust was a violation of their human rights as set out under articles 8 and 14. The Court of Appeal held that whilst Rampton was the claimants' home, it was not a private home but a public institution operated as a hospital under Section 4 of the 2006 Health Act which required all premises used by the public to be smoke free by 1 July 2007 (*R (E) v. Nottinghamshire Healthcare NHS trust and R (N) v. Secretary of State for Health*). Article 8 did not protect the right to smoke at Rampton. The dissenting judge Lord Keene held that the concept of personal autonomy which the Strasbourg court had adopted in *Pretty v. United Kingdom* was wide enough to incorporate a right to choose to smoke.

Right of health professionals to smoke

There is no statutory or common law right for a person to smoke as shown in the Rampton case (see above). Addicts may attempt to argue that articles 3 or 8 of the European Convention on Human Rights implicitly recognise such a right, but there is no decided case which has confirmed this right. (Article 3 recognises the right that no person should be subjected to torture or to inhuman treatment or punishment; article 8 recognises the right to respect for private and family life, home and correspondence, but there are many qualifications to this article 8 right.) Any such argument using article 3 would rest on the principle that to forbid a person to smoke was 'inhuman or degrading treatment or punishment' and therefore contrary to article 3. Alternatively, relying on article 8, the smoker would have to claim that the right of respect for private and family life included a right to smoke. However, the qualifications to article 8 include restrictions on the basis of the 'protection of health or morals, or for the protection of the rights and freedoms of others' which might defeat such an argument. The Rampton case illustrates the failure of an argument based on human rights in defending the right to smoke.

The registered nurse who wishes to smoke also faces a major hurdle as a result of the wording of the new NMC Code (Nursing and Midwifery Council 2008) which suggests that an extremely wide duty is placed upon the registered practitioner. It states that registered nurses or midwives must:

- *Work with others to protect and promote the health and wellbeing of those in your care, their families and carers, and the wider community.*
- *Provide a high standard of practice and care at all times.*
- *Be open and honest, act with integrity and uphold the reputation of your profession.*

Since it is now generally accepted that smoking is dangerous to health it could be argued that any nurse who smokes is failing to 'protect and promote the health and well being of ... the wider community'. He/she could also be seen as in breach of the requirement to act in such a way that justifies public trust and confidence. It could also be argued that a nurse who smokes is also failing to uphold and enhance the good reputation of the profession. It remains to be seen how the NMC will deal with any complaints about registered practitioners who smoke. The NMC includes in its draft standards for pre-registration nurse education requirements that the student should understand the concept of public health and the benefits of a healthy lifestyle and the potential risks of such behaviour as smoking.

Professional advice

The Royal College of Nursing (RCN) published a document, *Clearing the Air* (RCN 1999). It pointed out that smoking remains the single biggest avoidable cause of death in the UK and aims to increase nurses' knowledge of the impact of smoking on public health and support nurses in their role as providers of smoking cessation advice. In November 2000, the results of a joint *Nursing Times*, Department of Health and RCN survey showed that 90 percent of nurses who smoke wished to quit (RCN 2000). The joint initiative of these organisations, called 'No butts', aims to give nurses the practical information and support they need to give up. In 2000 the RCN published a self-help booklet (RCN 2000). The RCN welcomed the Department of Health strategy in February 2010 which aimed to reduce by half the number of smokers by 2020 and is taking active steps to support members in giving up smoking.

The Royal College of Midwives (RCM) joined forces with the Government in December 2001 to support pregnant women who smoke but want to give up (Department of Health 2001a). As part of this campaign, the RCM published an action guide for its members aiming to help midwives raise the issue of smoking with expectant mothers to improve the health of both women and their future children (RCM 2002). The Department of Health provided £3 million to fund the appointment of persons to co-ordinate antenatal and postnatal smoking cessation services. Sixteen medical staff resigned from Nottingham University in protest at its acceptance of a £3.8 million grant from the British American Tobacco Company to set up an international centre for corporate social responsibility (Wright 2001).The RCM has also collaborated with NICE in its guidance on smoking in pregnancy and after birth (see below)

Government policy

The Government has been pursuing a policy to encourage people to give up smoking and to support them. It initiated smoking cessation services in Health Action Zones in 1999/2000 following the White Paper, *Smoking Kills* (Department of Health 1998). There were three key targets: young people, adult smokers and pregnant women. The results of the first monitoring of these services were published in February 2000. In December 2001, the Government launched a new campaign, 'Don't give up giving up smoking' and encouraged potential quitters to ring the NHS Smoking Helpline (0800 169 0169) (Department of Health 2001b). In March 2001, the Department of Health announced that nicotine replacement therapy (NRT) would be made available on prescription, subject to consultation (Department of Health 2001c).

In April 2002, the National Institute for Health and Clinical Excellence (NICE) published guidance on the effectiveness of aids to smoking cessation (Department of Health 2002a). It advised that bupropion (Zyban) and NRT not only are clinically effective but also are among the most cost-effective of all health care interventions for giving up smoking. NICE estimated that the annual demand for NRT or Zyban in 2003 would be between 500 000 and 1.4 million prescriptions, costing the NHS between £20 million and £56 million (NICE 2002). The suppliers of NRT have agreed to give the NHS a rebate on their products once sales have exceeded a certain level. The Secretary of State for Health stated that this money will be passed to primary care trusts for stop-smoking programmes. *Improvement, Expansion, and Reform. – The next three years: Priorities and Planning Framework 2003–2006* which sets out a three-year plan for tackling smoking in the health service was published by the Department of Health in 2003 and is available from the Department of Health website.

In June 2010 NICE published *How to Stop Smoking in Pregnancy and After Childbirth* (NICE 2010).

The Department of Health has set up an NHS Free Smoking Helpline on 0800 0224 332 which provides information about the many services available to assist in giving up smoking.

Anti-smoking legislation

The Tobacco Advertising and Promotion Act 2002 banning press and billboard advertising of tobacco products in the UK came into force on 14 February 2003 (Department of Health 2002b), and provisions prohibiting sponsorship of sporting and other events by tobacco companies have been brought into force subsequently (Department of Health 2003a). On 30 September 2003 new warnings about the dangers of smoking became compulsory on every cigarette packet (Department of Health 2003b). An agreement between the Government and major suppliers of smoking cessation products enabled primary care trusts to give out free nicotine patches and gum (Department of Health 2003c).

Health Act 2006

The Health Act 2006 made provision for the banning of smoking in public places which included workplaces. A workplace must be smoke-free if more than one person works there (even if the persons who work there do so at different times, or only intermittently), or where members of the public might attend for the purpose of seeking or receiving goods or services from the person or persons working there (even if members of the public are not always present). The rules relating to smoke-free premises came into effect on 1 July 2007. Power was given to the Secretary of State to change the age of persons lawfully able to purchase tobacco and in July 2007 only those over 18 years were legally able to purchase tobacco products. The Department of Health estimated that 40000 people had given up smoking in the year following the prohibition on smoking in public places.

Evidence that a ban on smoking in public places can improve health is seen from evidence of its effects in the American town of Helena (*The Times* 2003). Smoking in public places was banned for six months and researchers showed that in comparison with earlier figures, the ban led to a 60 percent reduction in heart attacks. The ban was lifted after a legal challenge.

Application of the law to *Scenario 22.1*

The employer of the community nurse has a duty to take reasonable care of the health and safety of its employees. Once senior managers have been informed of the harmful environment within which the nurse is expected to work, they should take all the appropriate action to encourage the patient not to smoke when the nurse is present, and to ventilate the room before she arrives. Sharing the visiting of that person amongst the community nurses would also seem to be reasonable action to take. The prohibition on smoking in public places would not help the nurse since, although the patient's home is part of her working environment, from his point of view it is a private place. A person who suffered from asthma was awarded £17000 by an employment tribunal in an unfair dismissal action. She said that she had become ill in her first week at a community centre while working as an administrator in a room where smoking was allowed. She complained and was moved to the no-smoking reception area but the centre failed to enforce the no-smoking rule. Her boss smoked in front of her during an appraisal interview whilst she was telling him of her problems of working in a smoky environment (de Bruxelles 2003)

Conclusion

A cultural change has taken place over the last 10 to 20 years in relation to smoking. Smoking is now banned in public places and all employers should have introduced a no-smoking policy. The smoking ban also includes hospitals, and the patients in a special hospital have lost their legal challenge against a smoking ban. The emphasis is now on assisting individuals to give up smoking. Smoking is still one of the major contributors to death and disease and employers have clear responsibilities to support employees in giving up smoking and those who wish to work in a smoke-free environment. The Trade Union Congress, the anti-smoking group ASH and the Chartered Institute of Environmental Health published a report, *A killer on the Loose* (Trade Union Congress 2003) claiming that passive smoking at work kills three people every day and calling upon the Government to implement the Health and Safety Commission's Code of Practice which would ban smoking from the vast majority of workplaces. This has now been achieved but, ultimately, it is for each individual smoker to see the benefits of and get the help available for giving up. It is hoped that figures for smoking-related diseases will show significant improvements with the effect of the prohibition of smoking in public places and with individuals giving up.

References

de Bruxelles S (2003) Boss smoked in front of asthmatic. *The Times* 11 October

Department of Health website: www.dh.gov.uk/planning2003-2006/index.htm

Department of Health (1998) *Smoking Kills — A White Paper on Tobacco*. The Stationery Office, London

Department of Health (2001a) *Midwives and Government Join Forces to Offer Support to Pregnant Women who Smoke*. Press release. Department of Health, London

Department of Health (2001b) *Government launches new 'Don't give up giving up smoking'*. Press release. Department of Health, London

Department of Health (2001c) *Nicotine replacement therapy products to be available on prescription and general sale*. Press release, Department of Health, London

Department of Health (2002a) *Government's approach to helping smokers to quit is backed by new NICE guidance*. Press release. Department of Health, London

Department of Health (2002b) *The countdown starts on banning tobacco advertising and promotion*. Press release. Department of Health, London

Department of Health (2003a) *Tobacco advertising ban starts Friday*. Press Release. Department of Health, London

Department of Health (2003b) *New Cigarette packets warnings become law from today*. Press Release 30 September. Department of Health, London

Department of Health (2003c) *Ground breaking deal to help smokers quit*. Press Release 12 November. Department of Health, London

Dimond B (1996) Smoking mothers' rights and the maternity department. *Modern Midwife* 6(6): 10–11

Hawkes N (2002) Anti-tobacco campaigns to use USA shock tactics. *The Times* 21 November

HSC (2000) *Passive Smoking at Work*. The Stationery Office, London

Lister S (2003) Dead smoker's testimony starts tobacco test case. *The Times* 8 October

McTear v. Imperial Tobacco Ltd [2005] Scots CS CSOH 69(2) 31 May 2005

NICE (2002) *Guidance on the Use of Nicotine Replacement Therapy (NRT) and Bupropion for Smoking Cessation*. NICE, London

NICE (2010) *How to Stop Smoking in Pregnancy and After Childbirth. Public Health Guidance 26*. Available from www.nice.org.uk

Nursing and Midwifery Council (2008) *The Code. Standards of Conduct, Performance and Ethics*. NMC, London

Pretty v. United Kingdom (2002) 35 EHRR 1

R (E) v. Nottinghamshire Healthcare NHS trust and R (N) v. Secretary of State for Health The Times Law Report 10 August 2009

Royal College of Midwives (2002) *Helping Women Stop Smoking: A Guide for Midwives*. RCM, London

Royal College of Nursing (1999) *Clearing the Air: A Nurse Guide to Smoking and Tobacco Control*. RCN, London

Royal College of Nursing (2000) *How to Stop Smoking*. RCN, London

Trade Union Congress (2003) *A Killer on the Loose*. TUC, ASH and Chartered Institute Environmental Health, London

The Times (2003) Smoking ban 'boosts health'. News item. *The Times* 2 April

Wright O (2001) University cancer staff quit over tobacco aid. *The Times* 12 June: 6

CHAPTER 23

Whistle-blowing

> ### Scenario 23.1. Blowing the whistle
>
> Dave worked in the intensive care unit and was concerned at the staffing levels. On several occasions over a weekend he had been compelled to look after more than one ventilated patient at the same time and he feared that a serious tragedy was imminent. What action could he take?

Introduction

This chapter considers the statutory protection under the Public Interest Disclosure Act 1998 which is given to those who bring concerns of dangers and crimes to the attention of others, and are known as whistle-blowers. There have been concerns that in the past, nurses and other registered health practitioners have failed to draw attention to serious deficiencies in their organisations. Even when attention has been drawn, staff have felt powerless if no action has been taken by senior management and known dangers are allowed to continue.

Whistle-blowing

'Whistle-blowing' is the term which refers to the action of a person (usually an employee) who draws attention to concerns which have health and safety or criminal implications. The need to establish statutory protection for employees who raise concerns led to the passing of the Public Interest Disclosure Act 1998.

Public Interest Disclosure Act 1998

The Public Interest Disclosure Act 1998 received Royal assent on 2 July 1998 and came into force on 2 July 1999. It introduced amendments to the Employment Rights Act 1996. The explanatory memorandum envisaged that the Act would protect workers who disclose information about certain types of matters from being dismissed or penalised by their employers. The Act applies to specific disclosures which are shown in *Box 23.1*.

> ## Box 23.1. Protected disclosures under the Public Interest Disclosure Act 1998
>
> - That a criminal offence has been committed, is being committed or is likely to be committed
> - That a person has failed, is failing or is likely to fail to comply with any legal obligation to which he/she is subject
> - That a miscarriage of justice has occurred, is occurring or is likely to occur
> - That the health or safety of any individual has been, is being or is likely to be endangered
> - That the environment has been, is being or is likely to be damaged
> - That information tending to show any matter falling within any one of the above has been, is being or is likely to be deliberately concealed

To qualify for protection when one of the situations in *Box 23.1* is present, the worker making the disclosure must make the disclosure to his/her employer or to another person to whom the failure relates or who has legal responsibility, and be making the disclosure in good faith. Protected disclosures include disclosures made to obtain legal advice, and disclosures to a Minister of the Crown if the employee's employer is appointed by the Crown.

The Secretary of State has the power to make an order identifying other organisations or persons to whom a protected disclosure could be made, provided that the employee makes it in good faith and reasonably believes that any allegations are substantially true. Persons to whom a disclosure could be lawfully made are known as 'prescribed persons' and were listed in the Schedule to the Statutory Instrument. More persons were added to the list of prescribed person by amending regulations in 2003 and 2010 and are shown in *Box 23.2* (Public Interest Disclosure Order).

Other disclosures are protected, subject to specified conditions. These disclosures would include disclosures to the press, police, media, and MPs. The specified conditions for these disclosures are shown in *Box 23.3*. The fifth condition, as set out in *Box 23.4*, 'Satisfies one of the conditions set out in 43G(2)', includes the belief by the worker that he would be subjected to a detriment by his employer if he were to make the disclosure to him or the Secretary of State, and fears that evidence will be concealed or destroyed or that he has previously made a disclosure of substantially the same information to his employer. The reasonableness of the employee's actions are judged in relation to the factors set out in *Box 23.4*.

Box 23.2. Persons to whom disclosures can be made

Audit Commission	Certification Officer
Charity Commissioners	Criminal Cases Review Commission
Civil Aviation Authority	Commissioners of the Inland Revenue
Auditor General	Environment Agency
Food Standards Agency	General Social Care Council (to be replaced)
Care Council for Wales	Health and Safety Executive
Housing Corporation	Local Authorities
Information Commissioner	Care Quality Commission
National Assembly for Wales	Pensions Regulator

• The persons to whom a protected disclosure can be made can be found on the Public Concern at Work website – Prescribed regulators for England, Scotland and Wales.

Box 23.3. Conditions for certain specific disclosures

The worker:
• Makes the disclosure in good faith
• Reasonably believes that the information disclosed, and any allegation contained in it, are substantially true
• Does not make it for personal gain
• Satisfies one of the conditions set out in 43G(2)
• In all the circumstances of the case, it is reasonable for him/her to make the disclosure (see *Box 23.4*)

Box 23.4. Factors by which the reasonableness of the employee's actions are judged

• To whom the disclosure was made
• The seriousness of the relevant failure
• Whether the disclosure was made in breach of a duty of confidentiality
• Any action the employer or other person could have taken when first notified
• Whether the worker followed the procedure

Disclosures of exceptionally serious nature

When the failure is of an exceptionally serious nature, then it will be a protected disclosure if:

- The worker makes the disclosure in good faith.
- Believes it to be substantially true.
- Does not make it for personal gain.
- In all the circumstances it is reasonable for him/her to make the disclosure.

Protection

The protection given by the legislation is that a person who makes a protected disclosure and follows the correct procedure is protected from dismissal and from being subjected to other detriments. He/she could complain to an employment tribunal that his/her rights have been breached.

Gagging clauses

Any provision in an agreement between employer and worker is void if it purports to preclude the worker from making a protected disclosure.

Guidance from the Department of Health

Guidance has been issued by the Department of Health which requires every NHS trust and health authority to have in place local policies and procedures which comply with the provisions of the 1998 Act (Department of Health 1999). In 2010 the Secretary of State wrote a foreword to a guide on whistle-blowing compiled by the Social Partnership Forum and Public Concern at work called *Speak Up For a Healthy NHS: How to implement and review whistle-blowing arrangements in your organization*. ACAS has also prepared guidance on whistle-blowing in its A to Z list of advice.

Implementation of the Public Interest Disclosure Act 1998

In one of the first cases to be reported after the Act came into force, compensation of more than a quarter of a million pounds was awarded (Booth 2000). An accountant who was dismissed after blowing the whistle on his managing director's expenses claims was awarded compensation of £293 441 by an employment tribunal. The tribunal held that he was victimised by his employers for raising genuine concerns. The company announced its intention to appeal. A report by the charity, Public Concern at Work, stated that 1200 claims were made in the first three years of the whistle-blowing law and compensation of £10 million is being awarded every year (Gibb 2003) by employment tribunals to employees. The average payout was £100 000 and the largest, £805 000, was to a city worker who raised the alarm about illegal deals. A total of £30 million was paid out in the first three years of claims under the Act and this did not include claims which were settled without tribunal hearings.

Procedure to be followed in cases of dismissal in a whistle-blowing situation

The Court of Appeal has given a ruling about the process which should be followed where an employee alleges that he has been dismissed for making a protective disclosure (i.e. the employee was a whistle-blower). The facts of the case (*Bladon v. ALM Medical Services Ltd* 2002) were that B (Bladon) was employed as a charge nurse in a nursing home run by ALM. He was dismissed following disclosures made by him to a nursing home inspectorate on standards of care at the home. An employment tribunal found that B was unfairly dismissed because B had made a protected disclosure. However, the employment tribunal had refused to admit certain evidence which ALM wished to produce to rebut the contention that B was dismissed because of the protected disclosure.

The Court of Appeal held that where an employee complained that he had been dismissed by reason of his having made a 'protected disclosure', the employment tribunal should hold a directions hearing in order to identify the issues and ascertain what evidence the parties intended to call. The tribunal had a duty to allow the employer to adduce evidence challenging the employee's evidence before deciding those issues.

Good faith

In order to obtain protection under the Public Information Disclosure Act the employee must act in good faith. This term 'good faith' has been the subject of several judicial rulings.

In the Employment Appeal Tribunal, Julian Dobson successfully defended his wife's Public Interest Disclosure Act victory against the novel argument that even though she had been acting in good faith when she reported child abuse, she should lose as the employer had not believed her good faith at the time it dismissed her (*Mama East African Women's Group, Trustees of v. Dobson* [2005]).

The High Court ruled that a BBC broadcast, prompted by a whistle-blower's disclosure, that criticised senior managers at an NHS Trust for manipulating waiting lists was true in substance and not libellous (*Henry v. British Broadcasting Corporation (2)* [2005]).

Post-employment victimisation

The Court of Appeal ruled in *Woodward v. Abbey National Plc* [2006] that Public Interest Disclosure Act protection applies to post-employment victimisation. This is intended to discourage employers from trying to make things difficult for a whistle-blower after he has left by denying him a reference. The decision restates that the Public Interest Disclosure Act should be viewed as anti-discrimination legislation.

Compensation for detriment

In the Court of Appeal of *Melia v. Magna Kansei Ltd.* [2005], Adrian Melia represented himself and won his case that he should be compensated for the distress suffered and legal costs incurred until the date he resigned following his victimisation for whistle-blowing.

Details of many other cases are available on the Public Concern at Work website (www.pcaw.org.uk)

NHS case

A case was brought by a dismissed NHS employee, Ian Perkin, a former finance director at a London hospital, who alleged that he was dismissed because he exposed an alleged fiddle over cancelled operations. He lost his internal appeal against dismissal and the employment tribunal found him to have been unfairly dismissed, but had the procedure been appropriately followed it would have been a fair dismissal. They found him 100 percent responsible and no award was made. His appeal to the Employment Appeal Tribunal failed as did his appeal to the Court of Appeal (*Perkins v. St George's Healthcare NHS Trust* [2005]).

Criminal actions by health staff

Following the offences by Beverly Allitt, the Clothier Inquiry made several recommendations to detect the possibility of personality disorder in applicants for nursing posts, to set up procedures for management referrals to occupational health and to clarify the criteria for the triggering of such referrals (Clothier et al 1994). There would therefore be a duty on any employee who suspects that a colleague is acting suspiciously to advise the appropriate manager. The Clothier recommendations were reinforced by an inquiry chaired by Richard Bullock following the case of Amanda Jenkinson, a Nottinghamshire nurse who was jailed for harming a patient (Bullock et al 1997). The Government has accepted the recommendations that all NHS staff will have a pre-employment health assessment. Information provided to occupational health staff will remain confidential unless disclosure is necessary because a member of staff is considered to be a danger to patients, other staff or him/herself. In these circumstances there should be disclosure to the appropriate person or authority.

The Shipman case

Following the conviction of Dr Shipman for 15 murders an Inquiry was set up under the chairmanship of Dame Janet Smith DBE. The first report (Shipman Inquiry First Report) considered how many patients Shipman killed, the means employed and the period over which the killings took place. The second report examined the conduct of the police investigation into Shipman that took place in March 1998 and failed to uncover his crimes (Shipman Inquiry Second Report). The third report (Shipman Inquiry Third Report) considered the present system for death and cremation certification and for the investigation of deaths by coroners, together with the conduct of those who had operated those systems in the aftermath of the deaths of Shipman's victims. The report noted that the present system of death and cremation certification failed to detect that Shipman had killed any of his 215 victims. Even though many of the deaths occurred suddenly and unexpectedly and should under the present procedures have been reported to the coroner, Shipman managed to avoid any coronial investigation in all but two of the cases in which he had killed. He did this by claiming to be in a position to certify the cause of death and by persuading relatives that no autopsy (and therefore no referral to the coroner) was necessary. Even in the two deaths which were examined by the coroner, there was an inadequate investigation which failed to uncover the truth. No death of a victim of Shipman was subject to an inquest until after his conviction. The present system therefore failed to protect the public. The Fourth Shipman Report which was published in July 2004 considered the regulation of controlled drugs in the community.

Fifth Shipman Report

The Fifth Report was published in December 2004. It considered the handling of complaints against GPs, the raising of concerns about GPs, the procedures of the General Medical Council and the revalidation of doctors, and makes significant recommendations for the more effective regulation of GPs. It also made suggestions on the meaning of 'good faith', the requirement to demonstrate 'reasonable belief' and the nature of making a disclosure in a small workplace (such as a GP practice). It recommended that:

> There should be some provision (probably a telephone helpline) to enable any person, whether working within health care or not, to obtain advice about the best way to raise a concern about a health care matter and about the legal implications of doing so. ....This should be provided on a national basis.

No recommendations were made as to the means by which this telephone helpline should be provided.

The Sixth and final Shipman Report considered how many patients Shipman killed during his career as a junior doctor at Pontefract General Infirmary and in his time at Hyde. All the reports are available on line: www.the-shipman-inquiry. org.uk/reports.asp.

Appointment of medical and dental staff

On 1 June 2000, the NHS Executive issued a circular giving guidelines on the procedures to be followed in the appointment of hospital and community medical and dental staff (Department of Health 2000). Trusts were required to include in application forms by 31 July 2000 a declaration to be completed by the applicant (including locums) on whether or not they have been the subject of fitness to practice proceedings here or abroad and whether they have been the subject of a criminal investigation here or abroad. (The guidance was prompted by the discovery that a doctor who was guilty of professional misconduct in relation to a woman had been struck off the professional register in Canada 15 years before.)

Bristol report into paediatric cardiac surgery

Sweeping recommendations were contained in the report of the inquiry into children's heart surgery at the Bristol Royal Infirmary chaired by Professor Ian Kennedy (known as the 'Kennedy report') (Bristol Royal Infirmary Inquiry 2001). On 17 January 2002, the Secretary of State announced the action which the Department of Health was taking in relation to the Kennedy report. Both the full response and an executive summary are available from the Department of Health website (Department of Health 2002). The Kennedy report called for a climate of respect, openness and honesty. If its recommendations are implemented, those who are concerned about dangerous situations should find it easier to bring to the attention of management their concerns and ensure that the appropriate action is taken. However the NHS Redress Act (still to be implemented) did not include a duty of candour. The National Patient Safety Agency is pressing for more openness and reporting of incidents and near misses (see *Chapter 13*).

Public Concern at Work (PCaW)

Public Concern at Work is a leading independent UK authority on whistle-blowing which was established in 1993. It provides confidential advice to individuals who witness wrongdoing at work and are unsure whether or how to raise a concern. It describes itself as having four activities:

1. *We offer free, confidential advice to people concerned about crime, danger or wrongdoing at work;*
2. *We help organisations to deliver and demonstrate good governance;*
3. *We inform public policy; and*
4. *We promote individual responsibility, organisational accountability and the public interest.*

In 2008 it won a competitive tender to provide independent and confidential advice to staff, and policy advice to organisations throughout the NHS.

Its website is www.pcaw.org.uk. In 2010 it published with the Social Partnership Forum a guide on whistle-blowing entitled: *Speak Up for a Healthy NHS: How to implement and review whistle-blowing arrangements in your organization.* It recommends the following steps should be taken:

- Step 1: Read this document.

- Step 2: Gain commitment from the board.
- Step 3: Gain buy-in and leadership from the senior management team and senior clinical staff, and staff-side engagement.
- Step 4: Make the right start – policy, practicalities and consultation.
- Step 5: Brief and train designated contacts and managers.
- Step 6: Relaunch, communicate and promote.
- Step 7: Audit, review and refresh.

Its comprehensive guidance also sets out a concise explanation of the law relating to whistle-blowing. Case studies provide useful examples of whistle-blowing situations and their resolution. There is also a model letter to staff about their raising concerns within the organisation.

A report from the Parliamentary Ombudsman has strongly criticised the Department of Trade and Industry (DTI, now renamed the Department for Business, Enterprise and Regulatory Reform) for the 'inherently misleading' way it introduced new rules that prevent the public learning about whistle-blowing concerns raised under Public Interest Disclosure Act. As a result the DTI paid the PCaW charity £130 000 for misleading it and wasting its time.

Application of the law to *Scenario 23.1*

Dave should ensure that he has full details of the staffing problems in intensive care, with dates, patient numbers, and staff cover, including the skill mix, and that he puts these concerns in writing to managers with details of the actual and potential dangers. He should obtain a copy of the trust guidelines for implementing the whistle-blowing procedure and should follow this to the letter. If the manager fails to take action, then Dave should report his concerns to senior management. He must be acting in good faith, believing his concerns to be true. Ultimately, if there is a failure by his trust's board, chairman or chief executive to resolve his concerns, he would be entitled to report elsewhere. Useful organisations that may support him include the Care Quality Commission and the Health and Safety Executive. Also, he may find support from the Nursing and Midwifery Council which requires him, as part of his duties as a registered practitioner under its Code to take appropriate action when he has concerns about patient safety.

Conclusions

The Public Interest Disclosure Act 1998 gives protection to staff who act as whistle-blowers against dismissal and from suffering other detriments because they have raised protected concerns to others in accordance with the procedures. However, the legislation may be too heavy a tool to protect staff against more subtle discriminatory actions (appalling timetables, never getting leave when you want it, always getting the more unpleasant tasks in the department, etc.). To prove that these actions have occurred because of whistle-blowing may be difficult. Treating whistle-blowers fairly requires a culture within health care where there is a general concern to raise standards and to cease to protect those who present dangers to patient safety. If the new climate of respect, honesty and openness recommended by the Kennedy report is implemented, one of the consequences should be that 'whistle-blowing' becomes a quaint label of a historic and outdated past. The Department of Health published a consultation paper on a new NHS Redress Scheme (a statutory scheme of compensation for clinical negligence) and recommended that there should be a statutory duty of candour (Department of Health 2003). However the NHS Redress Act omitted such a duty and has not yet been implemented. It is clear that the NHS still has a long way to go in achieving a culture of openness and the work of Public Concern at Work and comparable organisations is still much needed in protecting individuals who become victims whilst raising concerns.

References

Bristol Royal Infirmary Inquiry (2001) *Learning from Bristol: The Report of the Public Inquiry into Children's Heart Surgery at the Bristol Royal Infirmary 1984–1995.* Cm 5207. July. The Stationery Office, London. Available from: http://www.bristol-inquiry.org.uk

Booth J (2000) Man who shopped boss wins £290000. *The Times* 11 July

Bullock R, Edwards C, Farrand I (1997) *Report of the Independent Inquiry into the Major Employment and Ethical Issues Arising from the Events Leading to the Trial of Amanda Jenkinson.* North Nottinghamshire Health Authority, Mansfield, Nottinghamshire

Bladon v. ALM Medical Services Ltd 2002 The Times 29 August

Clothier C, MacDonald CA, Shaw DA (1994) *The Allitt Inquiry: Independent Inquiry Relating to Deaths and Injuries on the Children's Ward at Grantham and Kesteven General Hospital During the Period February to April 1991.* HMSO, London

Department of Health (1999) *Public Interest Disclosure Act.* HSC(99)198. Department of Health, London

Department of Health (2000) *Appointment Procedures for Hospital and Community Medical and Dental Staff.* HSC 2000/019. June. Department of Health, London

Department of Health (2002) *Department of Health's Response to the Report of the Public Inquiry into Children's Heart Surgery at the Bristol Royal Infirmary 1984–1995*. January 2002. Cm 5363. DoH, London. Available from: http://www.dh.gov.uk/bristolinquiryresponsebristolresponseexecsum.htm

Department of Health (2003) *Making Amends. A Consultation paper*. Department of Health, London

Gibb F (2003) £10m for those who blew the whistle. *The Times* 30 April

Henry v. British Broadcasting Corporation (2) [2005] EWHC 2787

Mama East African Women's Group, Trustees of v. Dobson [2005] UKEAT 0219

Melia v. Magna Kansei Ltd. [2005] EWCA Civ 1547

Perkins v. St George's Healthcare NHS Trust [2005] EWCA Civ 1174

Public Interest Disclosure (Prescribed Persons) (Amendment) Orders SI 2010 No 07; and SI 2003 No 1993 (amending SI 1999 1549);

Shipman Inquiry First Report (2002) *Death Disguised*. Published 19 July 2002. Available from: www.the-shipman-inquiry.org.uk/reports.asp

Shipman Inquiry Second Report (2003) *The Police Investigation of March 1998*. Published 14 July 2003. Available from: www.the-shipman-inquiry.org.uk/reports.asp

Shipman Inquiry Fourth Report (2004) *The Regulation of Controlled Drugs in the Community*. Published 15 July 2004 Cm 6249 Stationery Office, London

Shipman Inquiry Fifth Report (2004) *Safeguarding Patients: Lessons from the Past – Proposals for the Future*. Command Paper CM 6394 December 2004 Stationery Office, London

Shipman Inquiry (2005) *Sixth Shipman: The Final Report*. January 2005 Stationery Office, London

Woodward v. Abbey National Plc [2006] EWCA Civ 822

CHAPTER 24

The future

There is no room for complacency in the NHS about health and safety. Across the range of areas covered in this book there are considerable challenges to be met in improving the safety of both staff and patients. In a report in 2003, the National Audit Office (NAO 2003) pointed out that staff sickness absences in the NHS were running at 4.9 percent compared with a national average of 3.7 percent for public administration, and the cost of this sickness absence was about £1 billion per year. Staff accidents and other health and safety issues, such as violence and aggression against NHS staff are major factors in staff absence. The NAO considered that whilst there had been some improvements since its report in 1996, progress overall was patchy. Moving and handling, needlestick injuries, slips, trips and falls and exposures to substances hazardous to health remain the main cause of accidents. It recommended that the NHS:

- Develops a national health and safety strategy to co-ordinate existing and new initiatives.
- Commissions and disseminates evidence-based guidelines on health and safety interventions to help the NHS trusts improve the management of risks and reduce the impact on stress, sickness absence and staff retention.
- Works with the NHS Litigation Authority and the Health and Safety Executive to support the development of a robust costing methodology for assessing the financial impacts/outcomes of accidents.
- Ensures that the new NHS Electronic Staff Records system is developed to capture information on reasons for work-related staff sickness.

In addition, the NAO recommended that NHS trusts:

- Should adopt a strategic approach to induction and other training and development based on an annual training needs analysis for all clinical and support staff.
- Review their strategies for providing occupational health services to ensure that they are proactive and cover key issues, including counselling, managing work-related stress, rehabilitation and other support for staff.
- Ensure better compliance and a more consistent and robust approach to

identifying, recording and reporting accidents, with measures for tackling under-reporting, drawing on the experiences of those trusts that have introduced good practice reporting systems.

Similarly, in its review of progress in the control of hospital-acquired infections and in particular MRSA, the National Audit Office concluded that implementation of its recommendations from 2000 was patchy and in the light of the increasing MRSA infection reports, much still had to be done (NAO 2004).

Many of these recommendations are being implemented, yet injuries from manual handling, and increases in the level of stress, bullying and violence all show that NHS managers still have a huge agenda in securing health and safety at work.

One of the difficulties faced by any health professional attempting to implement health and safety guidance is the complexity of organisations which are concerned with health and safety issues. A joint project between the Cabinet Office, the Public Sector Team and the Department of Health took place in October and November 2002 to reduce or remove unnecessary or bureaucratic burdens in the NHS caused by inspection, accreditation or audit. Its report was published in July 2003 (Department of Health 2003) and it was agreed that 55 actions would be taken to reduce the burdens and free up frontline staff to focus on health care standards and patient care.

Subsequently the Arms' Length Bodies Review (Department of Health 2010) which took place in 2010 has recommended fundamental changes to many of the NHS quangos which have been referred to in several chapters and are gradually being implemented.

Lord Young's Report: *Common Sense Common Safety*

In the light of the many concerns about our health and safety laws and procedures being too bureaucratic and cumbersome and causing too much red tape, the Government in 2010 appointed Lord Young to review the operation of the health and safety laws and the growth of the compensation culture (HM Government 2010). A summary of the recommendations in the report can be found in Appendix 1 to this book.

Many of these recommendations require legislation for their implementation and the Bills (detailed below) will be making their passage through Parliament in 2011.

HSE reaction to Lord Young's Report

The Health and Safety Executive (HSE) warmly welcomed the publication of Lord Young's Report into health and safety and stated that it was already working with others to develop responses to two of the recommendations: A 20-minute online risk assessment for offices (see below) with other web tools for similarly low-risk workplaces to follow and a new Occupational Safety Consultants Register (OSCR) (see below).

Judith Hackitt, the HSE Chair, said:

Lord Young's Report is an important milestone on the road to recovery for the reputation of real health and safety. HSE welcomes it and will be actively pursuing those recommendations within our remit.

We welcomed the review when it was announced by the Prime Minister in June and we are looking forward to contributing to its implementation.

Publication of the report is a tremendous opportunity to refocus health and safety on what it is really about – managing workplace risks. Getting this right is good for employers, employees and Britain as a whole.

We've been saying for some time that health and safety is being used by too many people as a convenient excuse to hide behind. Often it is invoked to disguise somebody's motives – concerns over costs or complexity, an unwillingness to defend an unpopular decision or simple laziness. Lord Young is sweeping these excuses away.

HSE will continue to champion a sensible and proportionate approach to dealing with serious risks in the workplace – not eliminating every minor risk from everyday life.

Online 20-minute risk assessment

In keeping with the aim to simplify health and safety laws, the HSE in 2010 announced that it was setting up a new online risk assessment. (HSE 2010). Its aim was to help cut back the time it takes to weigh up the hazards in offices to just 20 minutes. The Health and Safety Executive (HSE) states that it produced the web tool to help employers to consider relevant hazards in their office and think about how they control them to keep staff safe. The tool was aimed at helping to avoid unnecessary paperwork and bureaucracy for office-based businesses, which tend to be low risk. Safety officials would take account of the results of the assessments when they carry out inspections – evidence that businesses have taken appropriate steps to manage workplace risk.

Of this initiative, Judith Hackitt, the HSE chair, said:

Many people assume that risk assessments need to be long, formal documents covering every hazard, no matter how minor or unlikely to occur. That's not the case and the new 20-minute risk assessments make it clear that this can be done for any office quickly and easily. We've previously provided example risk assessments to help people identify the sort of risks they should be considering, but this goes one step further in helping employers actually do the assessment for offices. Employers know their businesses better than anyone – and with a little helping hand they can easily consider what is necessary to protect workers.

The HSE stated that complying with the law in a low risk business can be done with common sense by anyone. The online tool works by prompting employers to answer a series of questions about their workplace and then generates a unique risk assessment with actions required. The HSE already provides example risk assessments for 34 workplaces, including charity shops, estate agents and hairdressers. They help businesses get to grips with the sort of risks they will need to manage. The new 20-minute risk assessments differ because the online tool prompts employers to answer a series of straightforward questions that generates their risk assessment and action plan. Simplified risk assessments for other low risk workplaces are currently being developed.

The online risk assessment form can be found at www.hse.gov.uk/risk/office. htm

The Occupational Safety and Health Consultants Register (OSHCR)

Following another recommendation in Lord Young's Report, Health and Safety Consultants were invited to sign up to new benchmark register for health and safety on 31 January 2011. The new independent register is intended to become a new benchmark for standards in the profession. It aims to increase employers' confidence in accessing good quality, proportionate advice and also to address concerns that some employers, especially small and medium sized enterprises (SMEs), can find it difficult to know how and where to get external health and safety advice. OSHCR has been established by a number of professional bodies representing general safety and occupational health consultants across the UK, with support from the HSE. The register, which is voluntary, is open to individuals who provide commercial advice on general health and safety management issues and who have achieved at least one of the following: Chartered status with IOSH (Institution of Occupational Safety and Health), CIEH (Chartered Institute of Environmental Health), or REHIS (Royal Environmental Health Institute of Scotland) with health and safety qualifications; Fellow status with IIRSM (International Institute of Risk and Safety Management) with degree level qualifications; Member or Fellow status with BOHS (British Occupational Hygiene Society), or FOH (Faculty of Occupational Hygiene); Registered Member or Fellow status with IEHF (Institute of Ergonomics and Human Factors). In addition, all consultants wishing to join the register will be asked to declare that they will:

- *Demonstrate adequate continuing professional development;*
- *Abide by their professional body's code of conduct;*
- *Provide sensible and proportionate advice, and*
- *Have professional indemnity insurance or equivalent to cover the nature of their duties.*

The application process includes a check of an individual's membership status with the relevant professional body.

Speaking on behalf of all the organisations involved in developing OSHCR, HSE Chair Judith Hackitt said:

There are already many very good health and safety consultants who give sensible and proportionate advice to employers, but there are also those who may over-complicate health and safety, miss important hazards or contribute to misperceptions about what is really needed to protect people at work.

This register offers a level of assurance to businesses that those consultants on the register have met set standards within their professional body. It will be an independent way of demonstrating professional competence in occupational health and safety consultancy and should also encourage those who have not yet met these standards to do so.

The scheme is managed by the professional bodies themselves through a not-for-profit company, with the HSE providing support.

The application fee is £60, but applications received by 30 April 2011 were subject to a discounted fee of £30. The fee, which is non-refundable, covers the cost of processing the application and is payable annually on renewal of registration. Individuals who applied to join the register during the discounted period were given a registration renewal date of 30 April 2012.

To apply to join the register visit www.oshcr.org

Consultation on RIDDOR

A consultation on an amendment to the Reporting of Injuries, Diseases and Dangerous Occurrences Regulations 1995 (RIDDOR) was initiated in January 2011. The amendment was proposed by Lord Young in his report *Common Sense, Common Safety*. If adopted, the period of incapacitation after which an injury to a person at work must be reported to the enforcing authority, will change from over three to over seven days. The consultation sought views on the proposal itself and on the impacts that it would have if it became law. Under current rules when an employee is absent from work for more than three days following an incident, employers are required to report the injury to the relevant enforcing authority – either the HSE or the local council. The proposed amendment increases this 'over three day' period to over seven consecutive days. The change would align the incident reporting threshold with that for obtaining a 'fit note' from a GP for sickness absence, and would ensure that someone who has suffered a reportable injury has had a professional medical assessment. The consultation paper is available online at www.hse.gov.uk/consult/condocs/cd233.htm

The deadline for responses was 9 May 2011. The HSE will consider the responses and expects to submit recommendations to the Secretary of State for Work and Pensions.

Bills currently being debated in Parliament

As mentioned above there are many Bills now being considered in Parliament to implement Lord Young's recommendations. They include (descriptions of the Bills are taken from the Parliamentary website):

*   *Health and Safety at Work (Amendment)Bill 2010–11*: A Bill to amend the Health and Safety at Work etc. Act 1974 in respect of systems of risk assessment; to make provision for separate requirements for play, leisure

and work-based activities; to introduce simplified risk assessments for schools; and for connected purposes.

- *Health and Safety Consultants (Qualifications) Bill 2010–11*: A Bill to introduce qualification requirements for health and safety consultants; to provide accreditation for such consultants; and for connected purposes.
- *Low Hazard Workplaces (Risk Assessment Exemption) Bill 2010–11*: A Bill to exempt employers from the requirement to produce a written risk assessment in respect of low hazard workplaces and the premises of those working from their own home with low hazard equipment.
- *Reporting of Injuries, Diseases and Dangerous Occurrences Regulation Bill 2010–11*: A Bill to reduce the duties on employers to report matters under the Reporting of Injuries, Diseases and Dangerous Occurrences Regulations 1995.
- *Self-Employment (Risk Assessment Exemption) Bill 2010–11*: A Bill to exempt self-employed persons engaged in low hazard activity from the requirement to produce a written risk assessment.
- *Volunteering Bill 2010–11*: A Bill to make provision to promote volunteering; to enable potential volunteers to obtain a fit and proper person certificate for their activities; and for connected purposes.

Other Bills which have an impact upon some of the topics considered in this book include:

- *Apprehension of Burglars Bill 2010–11*: A Bill to provide immunity from prosecution or civil action for persons who apprehend or attempt to apprehend burglars; and for connected purposes.
- *Compensation (Limitation) Bill 2010–11*: A Bill to prevent conditional fee agreement success fees and after-the-event insurance premiums being recoverable from the losing party in civil litigation; to facilitate damages-based agreements for contingency fees in respect of successful litigants; and for connected purposes.
- *Consumer Protection (Private Car Parks) Bill 2010–11*: A Bill to make provision relating to the licensing of charging, publicly-available, privately-owned car parks; to require local authorities to introduce a licensing system for such car parks; to enable local authorities to recover the costs of such a licensing scheme from car park operators; and for connected purposes.
- *Consumer Protection (Postal Marketing) Bill 2010–11*: A Bill to make provision relating to the regulation of postal marketing; and for connected purposes.

- *Contaminated Blood (Support for Infected and Bereaved Persons) Bill [HL] 2010–11*: The purpose of the Bill is to provide support for people who have been infected with certain diseases as a result of receiving contaminated blood and blood products supplied by the National Health Service. The Bill would establish a compensation package for people who have been infected, their widows, dependants and carers. It would also set up a committee to advise on the treatment of haemophilia and a review into the support available for infected people and their families. Lord Morris of Manchester introduced a similar Bill with the same title in the 2009–10 parliamentary session. It completed its stages in the House of Lords on 21 January 2010, and received its first reading in the House of Commons on the same day, but made no further progress. Key areas:
  - All people with haemophilia who have received blood or blood products supplied by the NHS would be offered a test for hepatitis B and C, HIV, human T-lymphotropic virus, syphilis and variant Creutzfeldt-Jakob disease. Their partners would also be eligible to receive the test.
  - All blood donors would be routinely tested for these conditions, and donated blood would be subject to prion filtration.
  - People who have been infected by contaminated blood or blood products supplied by the NHS would receive NHS compensation cards entitling them to free-of-charge prescription drugs, counselling, physiotherapy, occupational therapy and home nursing, and priority NHS treatment whenever possible.
  - People who have been infected would be entitled to claim non-means tested financial compensation.
  - Widows and other dependants of people who have been infected, and those who have had to give up work to care for an infected person, would also be entitled to claim compensation.
  - A committee to advise on the treatment of haemophilia would be established. The committee would be involved in a review of the support available for people who have been infected by contaminated blood or blood products and their families.
- *Domestic Violence, Crime and Victims (Amendment) Bill 2010–11*: Section 5 of the Domestic Violence, Crime and Victims Act 2004 created an offence of causing or allowing the death of a child or vulnerable adult. The offence is limited to incidents where the victim died of an unlawful act and only applies to members of the household who had frequent contact with the victim. The household member must have either caused the victim's death

or failed to take reasonable steps to protect the victim, and the victim must have been at significant risk of serious physical harm. Only those who are 16 or over may be guilty of the offence, unless they are the mother or father of the victim. The Bill would amend Section 5 of the Act to widen its scope to include situations where children and vulnerable adults have been seriously harmed. 'Serious harm' is defined in the 2004 Act as 'harm that amounts to grievous bodily harm for the purposes of the Offences against the Person Act 1861'. The Bill would also make consequential amendments to Sections 6 and 7 of the Act.

- *Epilepsy and Related Conditions (Education and Health Services) Bill 2010–11*: A Bill to require action plans to be prepared for the provision of education and health services for children and adults with epilepsy and related conditions; to make provision about support for children and adults with epilepsy and related conditions; and for connected purposes.
- *Equality and Diversity (Reform) Bill 2010–11*: A Bill to prohibit the use of affirmative and positive action in recruitment and appointment processes; to repeal the Sex Discrimination (Election Candidates) Act 2002; and for connected purposes.
- *Fire Safety (Protection of Tenants) Bill 2010–11*: A Bill to require landlords to provide smoke alarms in rented accommodation; and for connected purposes.
- *Food Labelling Regulations (Amendment) Bill 2010–11*: A Bill to amend the Food Labelling Regulations 1996 to provide for information about the country of origin of food to be made available to consumers; and for connected purposes.
- *Mental Health (Discrimination) Bill 2010–11*: Make further provision about discrimination against people on the grounds of their mental health.
- *National Health Service Redress (Amendment) Bill 2010–11*: A Bill to amend the National Health Service Redress Act 2006 to facilitate faster resolution of claims and reduce costs; and for connected purposes.
- *NHS Acute Medical and Surgical Services (Working Time Directive) Bill 2010–11*: A Bill to require the Secretary of State to conduct an assessment of the impact of the European Union Working Time Directive on NHS acute medical and surgical services; to require the Secretary of State to make provision to exempt NHS acute medical and surgical services from the European Union Working Time Directive in the light of that assessment if certain conditions are met; and for connected purposes.
- *Rights Bill 2010–11*: A Bill to set out certain principles in a United

Kingdom Bill of Rights; to repeal the Human Rights Act 1998; and for connected purposes.

- *Road Traffic Accident (Personal Injury) (Amendment) Bill 2010–11*: A Bill to raise to £25 000 the upper limit for awards for road traffic accident personal injury claims introduced under the simplified claims procedure.
- *Safety of Medicines Bill 2010–11*: The Bill proposes the establishment of a Medicines Safety Evaluation Panel to compare the effectiveness of human biology-based tests and animal-based tests in assessing the safety of medicines. The panel would be required to report within two years and would have full access to all relevant records held by the Medicines and Healthcare Products Regulatory Agency.
- *Support and Protection for Elderly People and Adults at Risk of Abuse Bill 2010–11*: A Bill to promote awareness of abuse of elderly people and adults at risk, to promote training on how to recognise and respond to such abuse amongst those who are likely to encounter abuse in the course of their work, to promote greater awareness and understanding of the rights of victims of abuse amongst agencies with responsibilities for providing, arranging, commissioning, monitoring and inspecting care services, to promote the development of local strategies for preventing abuse of elderly people and adults at risk and for ensuring that victims are assisted in recovering from the effects of abuse.
- *Tribunals (Maximum Compensation Awards) Bill 2010–11*: A Bill to enable maximum limits to be established for compensation in tribunal awards for cases involving unlawful discrimination; and for connected purposes.
- *Young Offenders (Parental Responsibility) Bill 2010–11*: A Bill to make provision for a mechanism to hold individuals to account for any criminal sanctions imposed upon young people for whom those individuals hold parental responsibility; and for connected purposes.

It should be stressed that not all these Bills will complete their passage through Parliament and receive the royal assent.

Conclusions

Significant changes are currently taking place within the health and safety sector with a view to simplifying the legislation and ensuring that priority is given to actual risks as opposed to fanciful possibilities.

It is hoped that this book, by setting out the statutes, cases and official guidance and considering the practical situations which arise, will continue to be of assistance to all health service staff who have duties to promote the health and safety of themselves, their colleagues, their patients and the wider general public. This is a duty placed on each and every person individually.

References

Department of Health (2003) *Making a Difference: Reducing Burdens in Healthcare Inspection and Monitoring*. Department of Health, London

Department of Health (2010) *Liberating the NHS: Report of the Arm's Length Bodies* Department of Health, London

HM Government (2010) *Common Sense Common Safety*. Review by Lord Young. HMSO, London

HSE (2010) *20-Minute Risk Assessment for Low Risk Offices*. Available from: www.hse.gov.uk/risk/office.htm

National Audit Office (2003) *A Safer Place to Work: Improving the management of health and safety risks to staff in NHS trusts*. HC 623 Session 2002–3, 30 April 2003. NAO, London

National Audit Office (2004) *Improving Patient Care by Reducing the Risk of Hospital Acquired Infection: A progress report* HC 876 Session 2003–4, 14 July 2004. NAO, London

Lord Young's Report

Summary of recommendations

Compensation culture

- Introduce a simplified claims procedure for personal injury claims similar to that for road traffic accidents under £10000 on a fixed costs basis. Explore the possibility of extending the framework of such a scheme to cover low value medical negligence claims.
- Examine the option of extending the upper limit for road traffic accident personal injury claims to £25000.
- Introduce the recommendations in Lord Justice Jackson's review of civil litigation costs.
- Restrict the operation of referral agencies and personal injury lawyers and control the volume and type of advertising.
- Clarify (through legislation if necessary) that people will not be held liable for any consequences due to well-intentioned voluntary acts on their part.

Low hazard workplaces

- Simplify the risk assessment procedure for low hazard workplaces such as offices, classrooms and shops. The HSE should create simpler interactive risk assessments for low hazard workplaces, and make them available on its website.
- The HSE should create periodic checklists that enable businesses operating in low hazard environments to check and record their compliance with regulations as well as online video demonstrations of best practice in form completion.
- The HSE should develop similar checklists for use by voluntary organisations.
- Exempt employers from risk assessments for employees working from home in a low hazard environment.
- Exempt self-employed people in low hazard businesses from risk assessments.

Raising standards

- Professionalise health and safety consultants with a qualification requirement that all consultants should be accredited to professional bodies. Initially the HSE could take the lead in establishing the validation body for qualifications, working with the relevant sector and professional bodies. However, this function should be run by the professional bodies as soon as possible.
- Establish a web-based directory of accredited health and safety consultants.

Insurance

- Insurance companies should cease the current practice that requires businesses operating in low hazard environments to employ health and safety consultants to carry out full health and safety risk assessments.
- Where health and safety consultants are employed to carry out full health and safety risk assessments, only qualified consultants who are included on the web-based directory should be used.
- There should be consultation with the insurance industry to ensure that worthwhile activities are not unnecessarily curtailed on health and safety grounds. Insurance companies should draw up a code of practice on health and safety for businesses and the voluntary sector. If the industry is unable to draw up such a code, then legislation should be considered.

Education

- Simplify the process that schools and similar organisations undertake before taking children on trips.
- Introduce a single consent form that covers all activities a child may undertake during his or her time at a school.
- Introduce a simplified risk assessment for classrooms.
- Shift from a system of risk assessment to a system of risk–benefit assessment and consider reviewing the Health and Safety at Work etc. Act 1974 to separate out play and leisure from workplace contexts.

Local authorities

- Officials who ban events on health and safety grounds should put their reasons in writing.

- Enable citizens to have a route for redress where they want to challenge local officials' decisions. Local authorities will conduct an internal review of all refusals on the grounds of health and safety.
- Citizens should be able to refer unfair decisions to the Ombudsman, and a fast track process should be implemented to ensure that decisions can be overturned within two weeks. If appropriate, the Ombudsman may award damages where it is not possible to reinstate an event. If the Ombudsman's role requires further strengthening, then legislation should be considered.

Health and safety legislation

- The HSE should produce clear separate guidance under the Code of Practice focused on small and medium businesses engaged in lower risk activities.
- The current raft of health and safety regulations should be consolidated into a single set of accessible regulations.
- The UK should take the lead in cooperating with other member states to ensure that EU health and safety rules for low risk businesses are not overly prescriptive, are proportionate and do not attempt to achieve the elimination of all risk.

Reporting of Injuries, Diseases and Dangerous Occurrences Regulations 1995

- Amend the Reporting of Injuries, Diseases and Dangerous Occurrences Regulations 1995, through which businesses record workplace accidents and send returns to a centralised body, by extending to seven days the period before an injury or accident needs to be reported.
- The HSE should also re-examine the operation of the Reporting of Injuries, Diseases and Dangerous Occurrences Regulations 1995 to determine whether this is the best approach to providing an accurate national picture of workplace accidents.

Working with larger companies

- Undertake a consultation with the intention of having an improved system with an enhanced role for the HSE in place for large multi-site retail businesses as soon as practicable.

Combining food safety and health and safety inspections

- Combine food safety and health and safety inspectors in local authorities.
- Make mandatory local authority participation in the Food Standards Agency's Food Hygiene Rating Scheme, where businesses serving or selling food to the public will be given a rating of 0 to 5 which will be published in an online database in an open and standardised way.
- Promote usage of the scheme by consumers by harnessing the power and influence of local and national media.
- Encourage the voluntary display of ratings, but review this after 12 months and, if necessary, make display compulsory – particularly for those businesses that fail to achieve a 'generally satisfactory' rating.
- The results of inspections should be published by local authorities in an online database in an open and standardised way.
- Open the delivery of inspections to accredited certification bodies, reducing the burden on local authorities and allowing them to target resources at high risk businesses.

Police and fire services

- Police officers and firefighters should not be at risk of investigation or prosecution under health and safety legislation when engaged in the course of their duties if they have put themselves at risk as a result of committing a heroic act. The HSE, Association of Chief Police Officers and Crown Prosecution Service should consider further guidance to put this into effect.

Adventure training

- Abolish the Adventure Activities Licensing Authority and replace licensing with a code of practice.

HM Government (2010) *Common Sense Common Safety* A report by Lord Young. HMSO, London

Health and Safety Strategy of the HSE 2009

The health and safety of Great Britain: Strategy document

Foreword by Judith Hackitt CBE, HSE Chair

Our mission is to prevent death, injury and ill health in Great Britain's workplaces and we are seeking your support – for the strategy and by becoming part of the solution. The improvements in Great Britain's health and safety performance over the last three decades are already a collective achievement we can all take pride in – and build on. The 1974 Health and Safety at Work etc. Act and its underlying principles and philosophy provide us with a legislative framework that is adaptable and remains fit for purpose today. When the new Board of HSE formed in April 2008 we decided to take the lead in developing a new strategy, which would build on the many strengths of what we already have, but would also recognise the many changes that continue to take place around us and which present new challenges for the health and safety system as a whole. The consultation process has evinced widespread support for our approach from all stakeholders and has enabled us to fine-tune the strategy to take account of the views expressed. There is collective agreement that:

- We need renewed momentum to improve health and safety performance.
- We need to respond to a wide range of risks – from more small businesses, from new sectors and new technologies, as well as traditional industries and long-standing risks.
- We need to find new ways of engaging workforces in all workplaces of all shapes and sizes, using the knowledge we have gained from the past that properly involved unionised safety representatives achieved better health
- We need leaders who are committed to promulgating a common-sense, practical approach to health and safety in their own organisations and throughout the supply chains they work with, motivated by the real business benefits, not exemption from regulatory scrutiny.

- We need to regain the value of the brand for what is real health and safety and challenge its devaluation as a synonym for unnecessary bureaucracy and an excuse for not doing things. The strong co-regulator partnership between HSE and local authorities is integral to this strategy and to its delivery – but regulators cannot do it alone. We need everyone to play their part in delivering improved higher standards of performance in health and safety because it is delivery of this strategy that will count. We will measure and report our progress, but we should be clear that we will be measuring the success of our collective efforts, not just the role of the regulator. You have told us that you support our approach, now let us work together to make this a truly shared mission and to realise the many benefits. Prevention of pain and suffering to people caused by work is the major driver for us all, but doing the right things the right way also delivers improved productivity, increased workforce commitment and enhanced reputation. In a world that is continually changing around us, the need for us all to work together to make this happen is constant.

Resetting the direction

The Health and Safety at Work etc. Act 1974 established the simple yet enduring principle that those who create risk are best placed to manage it. The Act led to the setting up of the Health and Safety Commission (HSC) and the Health and Safety Executive (HSE) and established HSE and local authorities as joint enforcers of health and safety law. On 1 April 2008 the HSC and HSE merged to form a single entity known as the Health and Safety Executive (HSE). The HSE is the national regulatory body responsible for promoting the cause of better health and safety at work within Great Britain. It continues to work in close partnership with local authorities.

One of the first undertakings of the new HSE Board was to reset and reaffirm the direction of health and safety. This document presents the Board's strategy for the health and safety system as a whole. It recognises and addresses the many stakeholders who have a role in maintaining or improving health and safety standards. Those stakeholders include:

- Employers and their representative bodies.
- The self-employed.
- Workers and their representative bodies.
- The HSE.
- Local authorities.

- Government, through its departments and agencies etc.
- The devolved administrations and their agencies etc.
- Professional bodies.
- Voluntary and third sector organisations.

To be truly effective, health and safety has to be an everyday process supported by all as an integral part of workplace culture.

The pressures to improve

Great Britain has one of the best health and safety records in the world. However, although the rates of death, injury and work-related ill health have declined for most of the past 35 years, the rate of decline has noticeably slowed. Within the EU, considerable effort has been invested in raising standards and bringing consistency to health and safety legislation across all member states. Even so, Great Britain has the lowest average rate of work-related fatal injuries and only Sweden and Ireland have lower rates for non-fatal injuries resulting in the worker being absent for three or more days. Yet, despite the previous successes, today's headline figures indicate that the combined incidence of injury and ill health in Great Britain is much the same now as it was five years ago. Provisional figures for 2007/08 show that 229 workers were killed and 136771 employees were seriously injured at their place of work. Similarly, during the same period, approximately 2.1 million people were suffering from an illness reputedly caused or made worse by their current or past work. The emotional toll to families, friends and communities is enormous. Then there is the impact on the economy. Around 34 million working days were lost in 2007/08 due to the consequences of accidents at work and work-related ill health. Looking at the finances, it is estimated that the annual cost to society of work-related accidents and ill health is a staggering £20 billion (approximately 2 percent of GDP). Clearly, maintaining the status quo is morally, legally and financially unacceptable. The pressure is on to better understand why aspects of Great Britain's health and safety performance have apparently stalled, and to find ways of beginning again the process.

Everyone has a role

To bring about improvements in health and safety performance the need is for everyone to work together towards a set of common goals. For that to become a reality, each stakeholder within the health and safety system has to understand their role and become better at executing their responsibilities.

Employers, self-employed, manufacturers and suppliers

The Health and Safety at Work etc. Act clearly places responsibility on those who create the risk to manage it. This applies whether the risk maker is an employer, self-employed or a manufacturer or supplier of articles or substances for use at work. Whatever the corporate status, each risk maker has a range of duties that must be implemented to manage the risk.

Workers

All workers have a fundamental right to work in an environment where risks to health and safety are properly controlled. The primary responsibility for this lies with the employer.

However, workers have a duty to care for their own health and safety and for others who may be affected by their actions. The legislation requires that workers co-operate with employers on health and safety issues.

Third-party organisations

Representative organisations are in a position to play a key role in driving health and safety improvements. Some are already doing so. For instance, the TUC actively promotes health and safety, while many trade union appointed health and safety representatives do a commendable job in the workplace. There is also a good spread of employer organisations, trade associations, consultant firms and voluntary organisations providing health and safety guidance to members and clients. Plus there are other organisations such as Government departments and local authorities exerting influence throughout the supply chain by ensuring that contractors work in a safe and healthy way.

The HSE and local authorities

The HSE provides strategic direction and leads the health and safety system as a whole. In addition to inspection, investigation and enforcement, key activities include research, introducing new or revised regulations and codes of practice, alerting duty holders to new and emerging risks as they are identified, providing information and advice, and promoting training.

Local authorities operate in partnership with the HSE to ensure that duty holders manage their workplaces with due regard to the health and safety of their workforce and those affected by their work activities. To achieve this, local authorities, as with the HSE, provide advice and guidance on what the law requires, conduct inspections and investigations, and take enforcement action where appropriate. With regard to the public, there are many regulatory bodies whose remit includes protection of the public from work activities. Local authorities also have wider responsibilities for the safety of local communities. Where appropriate, the HSE and local authorities will therefore work with partner bodies to ensure that activities are co-ordinated, duplication of effort is avoided and that public safety is effectively delivered.

Our goal

- To investigate work-related accidents and ill health and take enforcement action to prevent harm and secure justice when appropriate.

Investigations and securing justice

The HSE and local authorities are independent regulators. Working in partnership, their primary focus is to assist duty holders in preventing work-related accidents and ill health. This is generally achieved through inspections and a range of proactive measures including stakeholder engagement, communications programmes and the provision of information and advice.

Investigating complaints, accidents and ill health is also an important lever for improving health and safety standards. In particular, the investigation of incidents is crucial to help determine the causes, learn and share lessons and ensure that necessary measures are in place to prevent recurrence.

Investigation also provides the basis for enforcement action to secure justice. Where appropriate, the HSE or the relevant local authority will rigorously seek justice against those that put others at risk and in particular where there is a deliberate flouting of the law.

Enforcement has three main objectives: Firstly, it seeks to compel duty holders to take immediate action to deal with the risk. Secondly, it promotes sustained compliance with the law. Thirdly, it looks to ensure that duty holders who breach health and safety requirements, and directors or managers who fail in their responsibilities, should be held to account for their actions.

Our goals

- To encourage strong leadership in championing the importance of, and a common-sense approach to, health and safety in the workplace.
- To motivate focus on the core aims of health and safety and, by doing so, to help risk makers and managers distinguish between real health and safety issues and trivial or ill-informed criticism.

The need for strong leadership

Health and safety leadership must start at the top. Whatever the nature of the organisation, whether in the public, private or not-for-profit sector, members of the board have both collective and individual responsibility for health and safety. As such, the need is for people of board-level status to champion health and safety and be held accountable for its delivery. Following the example of leadership at board level, leadership must also permeate throughout the management and supervisory levels and the workforce. In SMEs there should be at least one person committed to ensuring good health and safety performance. Health and safety leadership is all about accountability. It means taking ownership of risk and accepting responsibility for managing it. A health and safety leader is the person who drives cultural change by winning the hearts and minds of directors, managers, workers and contractors. A leader fundamentally alters the corporate ethos so that health and safety becomes 'the way we do business around here'. Importantly, good leadership maintains a focus on the real health and safety issues and distances itself from the 'jobsworth' approach and those instances where health and safety is used as a convenient excuse for not doing something.

Our goal

- To encourage an increase in competence, which will enable greater ownership and profiling of risk, thereby promoting sensible and proportionate risk management.

Building competence

It is important to understand that within health and safety legislation, organisations of all sizes are required to nominate at least one competent person to help them meet their duty to control the risks posed by their work activities. Larger organisations often appoint one or more members of the workforce to do this, while with SMEs the responsibility commonly rests with the owner/manager. Similarly, some organisations bring in specialist external consultants to help, and in other instances a professional body may be called upon to provide advice. However, in practice, legislative compliance should be regarded as the minimum acceptable standard. Truly effective health and safety management requires competency across every facet of an organisation and through each level of the workforce. The need is for health and safety training to place greater emphasis on coaching so that directors, line managers and workers alike are able to determine what is sensible and reasonable. Also, it is important that the education system embeds the basic understanding of risk as a life skill so that young people joining the workforce are more risk aware. The essence of competence is relevance to the workplace. What matters is that there is a proper focus on both the risks that occur most often and those with serious consequences. Competence is the ability for every director, manager and worker to recognise the risks in operational activities and then apply the right measures to control and manage those risks.

Our goal

* To reinforce the promotion of worker involvement and consultation in health and safety matters throughout unionised and non-unionised workplaces of all sizes.

Involving the workforce

Workplace research provides evidence to suggest that involving workers has a positive effect on health and safety performance. Equally, there is strong evidence that unionised workplaces and those with health and safety representatives are safer and healthier as a result.

The need is to develop a genuine management/workforce partnership based on trust, respect and co-operation. With such a partnership in place, a culture can evolve in which health and safety problems are jointly solved and in which concerns, ideas and solutions are freely shared and acted upon. In the first instance, training managers and health and safety representatives together will establish a shared perspective on tackling health and safety issues in their organisation and complement the training they already receive separately. This, in turn, encourages the combined involvement of management and health and safety representatives in inspections, investigations and risk assessments. Ultimately, the effect of workforce involvement is that operational practices and health and safety risk management are aligned for the benefit of all and with the co-operation of everyone. Whether unionised or not, no matter the size or scope of the organisation, worker involvement is fundamental to good health and safety performance and therefore to good business.

Our goals

- To specifically target key health issues and to identify and work with those bodies best placed to bring about a reduction in the incidence rate and number of cases of work-related ill health.
- To set priorities and, within those priorities, to identify which activities, their length and scale, deliver a significant reduction in the rate and number of deaths and accidents.

Creating healthier, safer workplaces

Central to the creation of healthier, safer workplaces is the need for all stakeholders in the health and safety system to set priorities. This applies whether the stakeholder focus is on an industry, a sector, a particular health and safety issue or an individual business or organisation. The starting point is to create a risk profile identifying which groups of workers are most at risk and the scale and incidence of injuries or cases of ill health. Bearing in mind the evolving nature of British society, care should be taken to acknowledge differences within the workforce in terms of ethnicity and language, cultural values and gender. Having a risk profile sets the priorities for health and safety improvement, which then enables resources and expertise to be more accurately targeted to deliver those improvements. With regard to work-related ill health, setting targets and implementing actions is complex. Some ill health is clearly work-related, albeit with long latency in certain cases. However, as every employer will recognise, other causes of ill health are not solely work-related or their seriousness may be exacerbated by non-work-related factors. In order to set health priorities and establish the most effective delivery mechanisms, collaboration is required to establish who should deal with specific issues. Key among those issues is how best to manage the interface between work and the other factors that may be impacting on a person's health. To make workplaces safer, in those sectors where injury has always run higher than average, the need is to find new ways of tackling old problems. Equally, in emerging sectors and those existing sectors energised by evolving technologies, the requirement is to recognise the inherent new risks and implement appropriate methods for managing them from the beginning.

Our goal

- To adapt and customise approaches to help the increasing numbers of SMEs in different sectors comply with their health and safety obligations.

Customising support for SMEs

Small businesses and other organisations make an important contribution to Great Britain's economic prosperity. However, they also account for a considerable number of the health and safety incidents reported each year. That is not to say that SMEs are inherently dangerous. Rather, it is the case that some SMEs conduct certain activities that carry a high level of risk. SMEs often find goal-based health and safety management difficult to apply. Therefore, the objective for the HSE, local authorities and all stakeholders involved with SMEs is to find new ways to help them understand how to comply with health and safety law in a manner proportionate to the risks posed by their work activities.

Our goal

- To reduce the likelihood of low frequency, high impact catastrophic incidents while ensuring that Great Britain maintains its capabilities in those industries strategically important to the country's economy and social infrastructure.

Avoiding catastrophe

Great Britain has a number of highly specialised industries providing products or services that are essential to contemporary living, such as energy for homes and workplaces and fuel to power vehicles. There is a risk though that if these industries are not properly managed they have the potential to cause harm to their workers and the public at large. Even a small failure in their health and safety regimes could have catastrophic consequences. Strong health and safety leadership is essential to make sure that the right systems are in place, that best practice is shared and that learning is disseminated from previous incidents. While recognising the economic and social importance of hazardous industries, the critical objective is to ensure that the hazards are kept firmly in check.

Our goal

- To take account of wider issues that impact on health and safety as part of the continuing drive to improve Great Britain's health and safety performance.

Taking a wider perspective

Health and safety does not and cannot exist in a vacuum. It is not a discrete entity and so Great Britain's health and safety priorities cannot be delivered in isolation from other issues that impact on or overlap with them. National legislation and its implementation has been and continues to be influenced by the EU. Similarly, Britain's socio-economic make-up and cultural values have changed enormously since 1974 and so the practice of health and safety must continually evolve to accommodate diversity within the population. From the Government's perspective, health and safety is just one part of the overall business regulation. Equally, for some years now, local authorities and many businesses have brought health and safety and other portfolios such as the environment together in terms of organisation and delivery. The reality is that health and safety integrates with a much wider agenda aimed at protecting people from harm and thereby benefiting not just the individual but society as a whole. This strategy seeks to continue improving the country's health and safety performance while recognising and responding to wider issues where it is appropriate to do so. As such, there is an acknowledged need for balance in managing the interfaces between health and safety and other law and also between the HSE and other regulators. Crucially, regulation must be a benefit to those it seeks to protect, not a disproportionate burden on those who have to comply with it.

Driving change for the better

The strategic goals for the health and safety of Great Britain are founded in common sense and practicality. They have one overriding aim: that is, to prevent the death, injury and ill health of those at work and those affected by work activities. The strategy is not asking for or expecting the impossible. Its essence is that everyone adopts a sharper focus on the priorities and takes leadership in addressing their responsibilities. The HSE is committed to directing its energies and resources to the achievement of the strategic goals. As such, it stands alongside all the stakeholders in the health and safety system and is prepared to be held accountable for its performance. The process of health and safety improvement began in 1974 and continued unabated until around 2003. Since then it has stalled. From now on, if all stakeholders work together with a clear vision and purpose, improvement can recommence and changes for the better can be realised. Ultimately, the goals set out in this strategy have four clear objectives for the health and safety of Great Britain:

- To reduce the number of work-related fatalities, injuries and cases of ill health.
- To gain widespread commitment and recognition of what real health and safety is about.
- To motivate all those in the health and safety system as to how they can contribute to an improved health and safety performance.
- To ensure that those who fail in their health and safety duties are held to account.

FURTHER READING

Bamber, L (2011) *Tolley's Health and Safety at Work Handbook*. 23rd edition Lexis Nexis, Butterworths, London

Barrett B, Howells R (2000) *Occupational Health and Safety Law: Text and materials*. 2nd edition Cavendish Publishing, London

Brazier M (2011) *Medicine, Patients and the Law*. 5th edition. Penguin, Harmondsworth

Chandler P (1999) *An A–Z of Health and Safety Law*. 3rd Edition. Kogan Page, London

Committee of Expert Advisory Group on AIDS (1994) *Guidance for Health Care Worker's Protection Against Infection With HIV and Hepatitis*. HMSO, London

Department of Health (2002) *AIDS/HIV Infected Health Care Workers*. Deparment of Health, London

Denis IH (2007) *The Law of Evidence*. 3rd edition. Sweet and Maxwell, London

Dimond BC (2010) *Legal Aspects of Occupational Therapy*. 3rd edition. Blackwell Scientific Publications, Oxford

Dimond BC (2005) *Legal Aspects of Midwifery*. 3rd edition. Books for Midwives Press, Hale, Cheshire

Dimond BC, Barker F (1996) *Mental Health Law for Nurses*. Blackwell Science, Oxford

Dimond BC (1997) *Legal Aspects of Care in the Community*. Macmillan, London

Dimond BC (1998) *Legal Aspects of Complementary Therapy Practice*. Churchill Livingston, Edinburgh

Dimond BC (2009) *Legal Aspects of Physiotherapy*. 2nd edition. Blackwell Science, Oxford

Dimond BC (2002) *Legal Aspects of Radiography and Radiotherapy*. Blackwell Science, Oxford

Dimond BC (2011) *Legal Aspects of Nursing*. 6th edition. Pearson Education, London

Gunningham N, Johnstone R (1999) *Regulating Workplace Safety: Systems and sanctions*. Oxford University Press, Oxford

Health and Safety Commission (1999) *Management of Health and Safety at Work Regulations*. Approved Code of Practice. HMSO, London

Health and Safety Commission (1992) *Manual Handling Regulations and Approved Code of Practice*. HMSO, London

Health and Safety Commission (1992) *Guidelines on Manual Handling in the Health Services*. HMSO, London

Howells G, Weatherill S (2005) *Consumer Protection Law*. 2nd edition. Dartmouth Publishing, Aldershot

Hurwitz B (1998) *Clinical Guidelines and the Law*. Oxford Radcliffe Medical Press, Oxford

Kennedy I, Grubb A, Laing J, McHale J (2010) *Principles of Medical Law*. Butterworth, London

Kennedy T (1998) *Learning European Law*. Sweet and Maxwell, London

Kidner R (2011) *Blackstone's Statutes on Employment Law 2010-11*. 20th edition. Oxford University Press, Oxford

Kloss D (2005) *Occupational Health Law*. 4th edition,. Blackwell Scientific Publications, Oxford

Malleson K, Moules R (2010) *The Legal System*. Butterworth, London

Markesinis BS, Deakin SF (1999) *Tort Law*. 4th edition. Clarendon Press, Oxford

Mason JK, McCall Smith RA, Laurie GT (2010) *Law and Medical Ethics*. 8th edition. Butterworths, London,

McHale J, Tingle J (2007) *Law and Nursing*. 3rd edition. Butterworth Heineman, London

Partington M (2010) *An Introduction to the English Legal System*. Oxford University Press, Oxford

Pitt G (2009) *Employment Law*. 7th edition. Sweet and Maxwell, London

Richards P (2010) *Law on Contract*. 9th edition. Financial Times and Pitman Publishing, London

Rowson R (1990) *An Introduction to Ethics for Nurses*. Scutari Press, London

Rowson R (2006) *How to be Fair in a Culturally Complex World*. Jessica Kingsley, London

Salvage J (1988) *Nurses at Risk: Guide to Health and Safety at Work*. Heinemann, London

Salvage J, Rogers R (1988) *Health and Safety and the Nurse*. Heinemann, London

Selwyn N (2011) *Selwyn's Law of Employment*. 16th edition. Butterworth, London

Selwyn N (2011) *Selwyn's Law of Safety at Work*. Law Society, London

Sime S (2007) *Practical Approach to Civil Procedure*. 10th edition. Blackstone Press, London

Tingle J, Foster C (2006) *Clinical Guidelines: Law, policy and practice*. Cavendish Publishing, London

Tschudin V (2003) *Ethics in Nursing: The caring relationship*. 3rd edition. Butterworth, London

Vincent C et al (1993) *Medical Accidents*. Oxford University Press, Oxford

Williams J, Vincent C (Eds) (2001) *Clinical Risk Management*. British Medical Association, London

Wilkinson R, Caulfield H (2000) *The Human Rights Act. A Practical Guide for Nurses*. Whurr Publishers, London

Zander M (2003) *Police and Criminal Evidence Act*. Sweet and Maxwell, London

WEBSITES

Audit Commission:
www.audit-commission.gov.uk

Bailii (case law and statute resource):
www.bailii.org/ew/

Bristol Inquiry (Kennedy Report):
www.bristolinquiry.org.uk

Care Quality Commission:
www.cqc.org.uk

Central Office for Research Ethics
Committees:
www.corec.org.uk

Civil Procedure Rules:
www.open.gov.uk/lcd/civil/procrules_
fin/crules.htm

www.justice.gov.uk/civil/procrules_
fin/index

Clinical Negligence Scheme for Trusts:
www.nhsla.com/Claims/Schemes/
CNST/

Council for Healthcare Regulatory
Excellence:
www.chre.org.uk

Department of Health:
www.dh.gov.uk

Domestic Violence:
www.domesticviolence.gov.uk

Equality and Human Rights Commission:
www.equalityhumanrights.com.

General Medical Council:
www.gmc-uk.org

Health and Safety Executive:
www.hse.gov.uk

Health Professions Council:
www.hc-uk.org

Hepatitis C website:
www.hepc.nhs.uk

Legislation:
www.opsi.gov.uk/legislation or
www.legislation.hmso.gov.uk

Medicines and Healthcare products
Regulatory Agency:
www.mhra.gov.uk

National Audit Office:
www.nao.gov.uk

National Health Service Litigation
Authority:
www.nhsla.com

National Information and Governance
Board for Health and Social Care:
www.nigb.nhs.uk

National Institute for Health and Clinical
Excellence:
www.nice.org.uk

National Patient Safety Agency:
www.npsa.gov.uk

NHS Direct:
www.nhsdirect.nhs.uk

NHS Institute for Innovation and
Improvement:
www.institute.nhs.uk/

NHS Professionals:
www.nhsprofessionals.nhs.uk

NHS website:
www.nhs.uk

NICE:
www.nice.org.uk

Nursing and Midwifery Council:
www.nmc-uk.org/

Occupational Safety and Health
Consultants Register:
www.oshcr.org

Office of Public Sector Information:
www.opsi.gov.uk

Open Government:
www.open.gov.uk

Parliamentary Publications:
www.publications.parliament.uk

Public Concern at Work:
www.pcaw.org.uk

Public Health Laboratory Service:
   www.phls.org.uk

Royal College of Nursing:
   www.rcn.org.uk

Royal College of Psychiatrists:
   www.rcpsych.ac.uk

Royal College of Surgeons:
   www.rcseng.ac.uk

Shipman Inquiry:
   www.the-shipman-inquiry.org.uk/
   reports.asp

Skipton Fund:
   www.skiptonfund.org/Eng

Stationery Office:
   www.hmso.gov.uk

UK Parliament:
   www.parliament.uk

Welsh Assembly Government:
   www.wales.gov.uk

World Medical Association:
   www.wma.net/e/policy/b3.htm

ABBREVIATIONS

ACAS	Advisory, Conciliation and Arbitration Service
ACOP	Approved Code of Practice and Guidance
AIDS	Acquired Immune Deficiency Syndrome
AvMA	Action Against Medical Accidents
CFSMS	Counter Fraud and Security Management Service
CHIP	Chemicals (Hazardous Information and Packaging for Supply) Regulations
CICA	Criminal Injury Compensation Authority
CLP	Classification Labelling and Packaging Regulations
CNST	Clinical Negligence Scheme for Trusts
COHSS	Control of Substances Hazardous to Health
CPE	Common Professional Examination
CPS	Crown Prosecution Service
CQC	Care Quality Commission
DH	Department of Health
DSE	Display Screen Equipment
DTI	Department of Trade and Industry
EMAS	Employment Medical Advisory Service
EPPs	Exposure-Prone Procedures
GMC	General Medical Council
HAI	Hospital-Acquired Infection
HASAW	Health and Safety at Work Act 1974
HCAIs	Health Care-Associated Infections
HIV	Human immunodeficiency virus
HPA	Health Protection Agency
HPC	Health Professions Council
HQIP	Health Quality Improvement Partnership
HSC	Health and Safety Commission (Merged with HSE April 2008)
HSE	Health and Safety Executive
HSMR	Hospital Standardised Mortality Ratio
IAG	Independent Advisory Group
ICC	Incident Contact Centre
ICT	Incident Decision Tree
IFL	Insulin for Life
JP	Justice of the Peace
LOLER	Lifting Operations and Lifting Equipment
LSCG	London Specialist Commissioning Group

MAC	Manual Handling Assessment Chart
MCA	Medicines Control Agency (Merged with MDA into MHRA in 2003)
MDA	Medicines Devices Agency (Merged with MCA into MHRA in 2003)
MHRA	Medicines and Healthcare Products Regulatory Agency
MRSA	Methicillin-Resistant *Staphyloccus Aureus*
MSD	Musculoskeletal disorder
MSM	Men having sex with men
NAO	National Audit Office
NCAPOP	National Clinical Audit and Patient Outcome Programme
NHSLA	NHS Litigation Authority
NICE	National Institute for Health and Clinical Excellence
NMC	Nursing and Midwifery Council
NPSA	National Patient Safety Agency
NQB	National Quality Board
NRL	Natural Rubber Latex
NRLS	National Reporting and Learning Service
NSF	National Service Framework
OSHCR	Occupational Safety and Health Consultants Register
PCaW	Public Concern at Work
PCT	Primary Care Trust
PPE	Personal Protective Equipment
PUWER	Provision and Use of Work Equipment Regulations
RCN	Royal College of Nursing
RIDDOR	Reporting of Injuries, Disease and Dangerous Occurrences Regulations
RSI	Repetitive Strain Injury
SACAR	Specialist Advisory Committee on Antimicrobial Resistance
SARS	Severe Acute Respiratory Syndrome
SME	Small and Medium Sized Enterprises
SMS	Security Management Service
SOPHID	Survey of Prevalent HIV Infections Diagnosed
SRSCR	Safety Representatives and Safety Committee Regulations
ULD	Upper Limb Disorder
WEL	Workplace Exposure Limits
WHO	World Health Organization
WRULD	Work-Related Upper Limb Disorder

INDEX OF CASES

INDEX OF STATUTES

INDEX OF STATUTORY INSTRUMENTS

INDEX